Alternative
Therapies
for PTSD

Alternative Therapies for PTSD

THE SCIENCE OF MIND–BODY TREATMENTS

Robert W. Motta

 AMERICAN PSYCHOLOGICAL ASSOCIATION

Published by
American Psychological Association
750 First Street, NE
Washington, DC 20002
https://www.apa.org

Order Department
https://www.apa.org/pubs/books
order@apa.org

In the U.K., Europe, Africa, and the Middle East, copies may be ordered from Eurospan
https://www.eurospanbookstore.com/apa
info@eurospangroup.com

Typeset in Meridien and Ortodoxa by Circle Graphics, Inc., Reisterstown, MD

Printer: Sheridan Books, Chelsea, MI
Cover Designer: Beth Schlenoff, Bethesda, MD

Library of Congress Cataloging-in-Publication Data

Names: Motta, Robert W., author. | American Psychological Association, issuing body.
Title: Alternative therapies for PTSD : the science of mind-body treatments /
  by Robert W. Motta.
Description: Washington, DC : American Psychological Association, [2020] |
  Includes bibliographical references and index.
Identifiers: LCCN 2020002001 (print) | LCCN 2020002002 (ebook) |
  ISBN 9781433832208 (paperback) | ISBN 9781433832215 (ebook)
Subjects: MESH: Stress Disorders, Post-Traumatic—therapy | Complementary Therapies
Classification: LCC RC552.P67 (print) | LCC RC552.P67 (ebook) | NLM WM 172.5 |
  DDC 616.85/21—dc23
LC record available at https://lccn.loc.gov/2020002001
LC ebook record available at https://lccn.loc.gov/2020002002

http://dx.doi.org/10.1037/0000186-000

Printed in the United States of America

10 9 8 7 6 5 4 3 2 1

CONTENTS

Alternative Therapies for PTSD

Introduction

We soldiers of the U.S. Army's First Cavalry Division are silhouetted from behind by a full moon. The year is 1971, and it is a typical hot, steamy, insect-infested jungle night. We are doing guard duty at an army encampment in Bien Hoa, South Vietnam. Armed with rifles, machine guns, and grenade launchers, we are positioned along a berm protecting our unit behind us. M18 Claymore mines, which explode in the direction of intruders, are laid in front of us and can be set off through hidden trip wires by anyone trying to sneak up on us. I am 22 years old, one of the elders in our unit, and college educated. Most are teenage high-school grads. Drafted into the army after graduating from college—and no longer protected by a student deferment—my sentiments are very much antiwar and anti-Vietnam involvement. Nevertheless, once in the army, I volunteer to go to Vietnam out of some misguided desire for adventure and to gain firsthand experience about war.

And then, at that instant in the still of that hot night, I hear something that sends fear to my core. I hear the unmistakable sound of someone crawling through the bush in front of us and toward our position. My heart is now racing unimaginably fast as I try to insert an ammunition clip into my M16 rifle. The full moon has lit us up from behind, making us easy targets. We are about to die.

We're trapped because we have been ordered to not fire our weapons without permission because of disturbing civilian casualties that have taken place. To fire so that we may protect ourselves and save our lives, we are required to call on a military field phone to headquarters and obtain permission.

http://dx.doi.org/10.1037/0000186-001
Alternative Therapies for PTSD: The Science of Mind–Body Treatments, by R. W. Motta

Whispering on a phone in the dead quiet of night would give away our position so that we would be even easier targets than we are now. I am desperately trying to insert that ammo clip into my rifle while keeping my head lowered, but I am shaking so badly that the action is almost impossible. I know and fear that a bullet from an enemy AK-47 assault rifle will, in the next millisecond, hit me straight in the head. I will die here. My intense rush of fear is soon accompanied by an overwhelming sadness and sense of disbelief:

> This is it. I'm going to die in this stinking jungle. Can this really be happening? I'm going to be delivered to my poor, poor mother in a green plastic body bag. What a waste of life, what a waste of a good education. How stupid, how wasteful, how sad! How could I let this happen to me by volunteering? Look what I've done.

Suddenly, gunfire erupts from somewhere. It is not clear. It is confusing. And then the night opens up with machine-gun fire, rocket-propelled grenades, grenade launchers, M16s, and AK-47 assault rifles. I am firing away with my M16 rifle, and then the clip is empty. I pick up a grenade launcher and start firing grenades in the direction where I heard the crawling. All hell has broken loose. A nightmare of unimaginable chaos takes hold. Total and utter confusion surrounds us. Rifle fire and explosions seem to be everywhere. And then, as often happens in these firefights, the shooting and the ear-splitting chaos slowly begins to subside, and we wait for the approaching dawn. We find nothing when the sun rises. There is no doubt that someone or something was out beyond our Claymores because they have been set off and exploded. We don't care. We are alive. We survived, and that is all that matters. We have survived one more day in what was euphemistically called the "Democratic People's Republic of South Vietnam." All I want is to go home, but I have gut-wrenching doubts that I ever will. I've aged years in one night.

The memories of this event and similar events are seared into my brain and will remain there until the day I die. The feeling of imminent death, of being trapped by our orders not to fire, and of the moon lighting us up for easy targeting is part of my being. It is part of who I am. I fear this kind of confinement, this life-threatening entrapment to this day. In that instant, on the verge of death, in that unbearably hot jungle environment, I was transformed from a naive antiwar activist into an animal. This newfound self, this animal, cared about only one thing: survival. This transformation is what posttraumatic stress disorder (PTSD) is really about, and it takes place regardless of whether the trauma involves war, rape, natural disaster, mugging, sexual abuse, the observation of horrific and deadly scenes, and many other overwhelming experiences. Fear and entrapment are critical elements of PTSD. PTSD transforms people in negative ways, and these transformations can last a long time, perhaps a lifetime.

As I write these words, I feel myself welling up with emotion. The memories of that night are as vivid to me today as they were more than 4 decades ago. These memories, these transformations of self, are why those with PTSD live both in this world and in a world they once inhabited. They lead a double life. They often feel like imposters in this world of laws, justice, and predictability. Part of them inhabits another world, an insane world of fear and chaos. Traumatic experiences are overwhelming, impossible to grasp, and totally negating of any sense of fairness, reason, or constancy.

Despite the altering experience I just described, I was one of the supremely lucky ones. I take no credit for not coming home in a bag. It was just luck. I came home physically alive but emotionally dead. I suppressed the trauma of war, went to graduate school, and became a psychologist, researcher, and professor. The director of the doctoral program to which I had applied, Julia Vane, told me that my application material arrived soiled by mud, given that it was mailed from what we referred to as "the boonies." To this day, I continue to carry the guilt in knowing that more than 58,000 Americans just like me did not come home alive. They came home in body bags, and it was simply the roll of the dice that allowed me, a volunteer, to make it home and do something with my life and help others. My personal experiences with PTSD and my research and practice have provided guidance in understanding and treating traumatized adults and children. I now direct a university-based trauma clinic for children and families.

THE SEARCH FOR ALTERNATIVE METHODS FOR TREATING PTSD

After many years of practice, research, teaching, and supervision, I've come to the conclusion that despite our well-intended efforts, there are serious problems with our ability to treat PTSD. I don't pretend to have the answers to what the best ways are to treat this disorder. Nevertheless, I am aware of the limitations of our current methods and am equally aware of the need for alternatives to traditional modes of treatment. My experiences in Vietnam and my professional experiences have served to provide guidance and understanding in treating the disorder of PTSD. I hope to share some of those insights in this book on alternative and complementary treatments for PTSD.

Like many who suffer the effects of trauma, I did not realize I had PTSD when I came home, and I didn't even know what PTSD was. My view was that I was a survival machine trying to pass as a hardworking doctoral student. My nights were filled with dreams of war and sleeplessness. The Fourth of July, as you might imagine, was a real problem and left me dysfunctional into the next day.

I coped with my unrecognized PTSD primarily by the method most traumatized individuals use: avoidance. I tried to not allow thoughts of the war enter my mind, and I immersed myself in my studies and drank to deaden the pain that my body was aware of but my mind rejected. This avoidance continued for years. And then, unwittingly, I benefited from a form of graded exposure therapy: confronting the trauma in little steps—in my case, by teaching and doing research on trauma disorders. I took up the alternative treatments advocated in this volume. Regular exercise, meditation, and yoga are among my tools. Yoga came last because I was not comfortable with the concept of uniting body and mind, and increasing the awareness of both. Lack of awareness and avoidance seemed to have served me well for many years. Unfortunately, avoidance is a short-term gain for a long-term loss strategy. In the short run, avoidance allows one to not deal with anxiety-provoking memories. In the long run, the memories and pain persist because the person has not dealt with them.

The thought of going for treatment at a Department of Veterans Affairs (VA) facility and being provided with cognitive behavior therapy (CBT), prolonged exposure therapy, and therapy groups was, and to some extent still is, too much to deal with. As a person who has experienced PTSD, I've chosen a gentler approach for myself, for my clients, and in our trauma clinic. These more tolerable approaches include some presented in this book as alternative therapies. They are primarily nonmedical alternatives to traditional psychotherapies. More directive and confronting approaches of traditional therapies most often lead to clients' becoming overwhelmed and fleeing therapy.

OVERVIEW OF THIS BOOK

I have selected the alternative approaches to the treatment of PTSD to include in this book because they meet three important criteria:

- They have been shown to ameliorate the symptoms of PTSD.
- They have amassed a degree of empirical support that allows them to not be considered the latest "fringe" method of treating problems.
- They do not place a heavy emphasis on reconfronting one's trauma experience in painful detail.

Although traditional therapies emphasizing the confronting again and processing of trauma experiences are considered gold standard treatments, they produce such a high level of avoidance among trauma sufferers that their utility is significantly compromised. Trauma therapists are often desperate to find effective approaches to treating PTSD that do not send their clients fleeing from therapy because of the extreme levels of anxiety that treatment often evokes. It is hoped that the approaches presented in this volume will become useful tools for clinicians and researchers in treating PTSD and in understanding the empirical bases of these methods.

Chapter Contents

Each chapter includes the following:

- overview of the intervention,
- description of the treatment process,

- case example,
- empirical research supporting the particular alternative intervention, and
- summary.

Chapter 1 attempts to give readers a succinct view of what PTSD is and how it often alters the self-view of the trauma sufferer. In addition, the critical role of avoidance, which is one of the diagnostic criteria of PTSD, is highlighted as a central factor that explains why trauma sufferers often stay away from traditional forms of psychotherapy. The anxiety that the traditional methods evoke often translates into quitting therapy. I review specific CBTs and address the need for alternative approaches.

Chapter 2 discusses eye-movement desensitization and reprocessing (EMDR). Although EMDR is now recognized as an empirically supported treatment for PTSD by many professional organizations, including the American Psychological Association, it continues to be viewed with suspicion and doubt perhaps because it does not fit into traditional learning theory explanations for why it works. Its methods and procedures bear few resemblances to traditional CBT treatment; as a result, the majority of therapists often reject EMDR, and academic and research communities especially shun it.

Chapter 3 covers yoga, which has become increasingly popular as a mode of intervention for those suffering from PTSD. It is likely that it is popular among trauma sufferers because yoga does not require anxiety-provoking recall and reprocessing of trauma experiences. PTSD often results in a separation of physical, emotional, and mental states, and yoga emphasizes and facilitates their integration. Trauma-sensitive yoga is a particular modification of yoga techniques that has been found useful in treating PTSD.

Chapter 4 presents mindfulness meditation as a discipline that trains individuals to focus on the here and now, and reduce ever present mind wandering. This training is particularly important for PTSD sufferers, whose minds are frequently drawn to painful recollections and images of their distressing experiences. Specific meditation techniques that enhance perceptions of control and tranquility include the mountain meditation, lake meditation, and the loving-kindness meditation. Overall, training in mindfulness improves one's control over distressing and intrusive thoughts as it enhances the ability to focus on the present and to produce tranquil states of mind.

Chapter 5 highlights recent findings on the unexpected value of physical exercise in reducing PTSD and accompanying anxiety and depression. Although it is unclear why exercise, and particularly aerobic exercise, is of value in reducing PTSD, research suggests that physical and mental states are inseparable and, as a result, physical exercise, by necessity, enhances emotional well-being. The chapter presents research showing PTSD reductions through exercise for children, adolescents, and adults.

The utility of natural environments and the presence of animals are addressed in Chapter 6, especially in regard to their utility in helping veterans and other traumatized groups with the management of their PTSD. Interacting with animals helps to develop a capacity to connect emotionally, and being in the presence of natural environments reduces the high anxiety and distress levels of those with PTSD. Dogs in particular have been specifically trained to ameliorate specific PTSD symptoms and are certified for that purpose.

Chapter 7 covers the use of acupuncture in treating PTSD. Evidence of the value of acupuncture in reducing pain is substantial, and the World Health Organization has endorsed acupuncture as a valid pain intervention. The chapter reviews recent studies demonstrating the use of acupuncture in reducing PTSD. Western medicine has no generally accepted explanation for the effectiveness of acupuncture, but Eastern medicine attributes its beneficial impact to the unblocking of the bodily and spiritual energy, qi (pronounced *chee*). Western researchers appear to be at a loss as to why acupuncture alleviates both psychological and physical distress, and yet it does.

Chapter 8 covers a relatively new alternative therapy for PTSD: EFT, or emotional freedom techniques. Rather than using needles as in acupuncture, EFT involves a body-tapping sequence that the trauma sufferer or client performs while making statements of self-acceptance and self-affirmation. The chapter details the mechanics of how EFT is done and also presents the empirical evidence, including meta-analyses, that support its efficacy in treating PTSD. Despite supportive evidence, EFT, much like EMDR, has encountered resistance from traditionally trained clinicians and researchers.

Chapter 9 reviews the use of 3,4-methylenedioxymethamphetamine (MDMA), which goes by the street name "Ecstasy," in treating PTSD. The effectiveness of MDMA for ameliorating trauma-related disorders is so compelling that the U.S. Food and Drug Administration has fast-tracked it for approval. Its primary impact is that it promotes feelings of empathy and compassion, and it allows PTSD sufferers to confront their traumas without undue anxiety. Given the large number of treatment-resistant cases of PTSD seen at VA medical centers, this labor-intensive treatment could actually prove itself economically viable in contrast to existing, often unproductive psychotherapeutic treatments that go on for years.

Chapter 10 provides a summary of strengths and weakness of all the alternative therapies for PTSD covered in this book. It also touches on other emerging therapies that have not yet garnered strong empirical support.

The Appendix provides readers with written, video, and other Internet resources that they may find useful for treatment planning and research. Given the ever-increasing numbers of people who suffer the cruel psychological impact of trauma and PTSD, the field is clearly in need of treatments such as those covered in this book.

Key Considerations for Alternative PTSD Treatments

Despite the value of these alternative approaches to therapy, which are sometimes referred to as CAM (complementary and alternative medicine) approaches, I don't believe one ever completely overcomes the impact of trauma just as one never really overcomes the impact of grief. Grief involves the loss of a loved one; trauma, the loss of the self. It is hoped that the approaches presented in this volume are helpful to those who are in the position to treat traumatized individuals and will serve as a vehicle through which those who have been traumatized can find a little peace.

CLOSING THOUGHTS

A telling occurrence is worthy of mention point. I recently bowed to the pressures of my wife and visited our local VA hospital after 47 years of having avoided the VA at all costs. Just driving there created so much anxiety that I was *dissociating*, that is, temporarily losing awareness of where I was going or why.

A psychiatrist interviewed me. It is difficult to put into words how troubling this interview was because intense emotions were the dominant theme during this meeting. I became highly upset when asked questions like, "Did you see dead bodies?" "Did you see dismembered or mutilated bodies?" "Did you shoot anyone?" "Did you feel you were going to die?" "Do you feel guilty that you came home and others did not?" "Describe your nightmares." To say this meeting was troubling is the height of understatement. I couldn't have fled that "mental health" office fast enough. The aversion I felt toward this directive, confronting style of interview bordered on extreme revulsion and energized the urge to escape as quickly as possible.

This traditional confronting approach, which is used in many therapies, creates such a level of aversion that most traumatized combatants, including me, stay as far away from the VA as possible. Alternative approaches to dealing with PTSD are clearly needed.

1

PTSD and Its Treatment

The impetus for this book, aside from personal experiences, evolved from a unique facet of posttraumatic stress disorder (PTSD), and this characteristic has made treatment of the disorder maddeningly problematic. In the current version of the *Diagnostic and Statistical Manual of Mental Disorders* (fifth ed. [*DSM–5*]; American Psychiatric Association, 2013), and in earlier iterations of the *DSM*, a central criterion for diagnosing PTSD is avoidance. An appreciation of the dominating and unique power of avoidance allows one to fully grasp the need for alternatives to standard treatments for PTSD.

PTSD AND TREATMENT AVOIDANCE

What is avoidance in regard to PTSD? It is simply a tendency to stay away from anything that reminds the sufferer of their traumatic experience. This avoidance, unfortunately, often includes therapy and therapists. The client suffering from exposure to trauma avoids sights, sounds, odors and all other sensations, perceptions, memories, and any other reminders of their trauma. This avoidance can be active, such as consciously staying away from an area of town where one was sexually assaulted. Or it may be unconscious, for example, getting lost while driving to a painful orthodontic procedure despite knowing the directions or, for a recently returned combat veteran, not being able to recall a just seen news story about a conflict between combatants. Avoidance is the most common way in which people deal with distressing

http://dx.doi.org/10.1037/0000186-002
Alternative Therapies for PTSD: The Science of Mind–Body Treatments, by R. W. Motta

situations. Of course, people avoid therapy for many other reasons, including scheduling issues, expense, and unwillingness to do the work needed to improve one's emotional state. Nevertheless, the influence of avoidance cannot be discounted.

The relevance of avoidance to psychological treatment of trauma is that most forms of treatment involve some form of recalling and going over the traumatic experience in detail. This decidedly painful revisiting of the traumatic past brings about an almost reflexive tendency to avoid the pain, which translates into the client's having second thoughts about the whole therapeutic process. Getting better often involves dealing again with the trauma in the form of describing what happened, how one felt at the time, and how one has managed subsequently. The process is so difficult that the client often cancels their session with the therapist or simply does not show up. Considerable literature indicates that when one confronts their traumatic experience either through procedures labeled as exposure therapy or cognitive behavior therapy (CBT), there's a good chance that their symptoms will diminish (e.g., Foa, Hembree, & Rothbaum, 2007; Foa & Kozak, 1986). What is not mentioned in this literature is that the majority of people who experience trauma would not even begin to consider going into therapy because they know they will have to discuss their experience, and this is the last thing they want to do. What they most desire is to put the experience behind them or have it somehow go away, or wish it had never happened. Unfortunately, it did happen, and often the painful memories, sensations, and perceptions persist. The memories of a sexual assault, of witnessing an adolescent's suicide, of losing family members in war, of fearing for one's own life in a genocidal attack, for example, can persist often to the end of one's days.

Why Do People Drop Out of PTSD Treatment?

No universally accepted and empirically validated answer satisfies this question, but the available research points to avoidance of trauma memories as being a significant factor contributing to dropout from PTSD treatment. In attempting to address the question of dropout, researchers and therapists are confronted with difficulties from the outset when we realize that the majority of people with mental health problems don't enter into therapy in the first place, and this is probably even more the case among those who experience the heightened anxiety levels associated with PTSD. When we examine high-quality experimental studies in an effort to answer why people drop out of PTSD treatment, we are often dealing with samples of people who have clear-cut symptoms of PTSD, are motivated to engage in research studies, are treated with strict treatment protocols, and are knowingly randomly assigned to conditions.

These people, however, frequently are not representative of the general population of trauma sufferers. Often those with PTSD who do not participate in studies may be homeless, may be drug involved, have a myriad of psychological problems in addition to PTSD, and may have low motivation to be treated or to participate in someone's research project. So, when we consider what the research is telling us, we must do so with an acknowledgment that we may be dealing with samples that are not necessarily representative of those suffering from PTSD (e.g., Zayfert et al., 2005). Research studies often are composed of volunteers who are motivated to participate. When those studies report the percentage of participants who dropped out of the study, that percentage is likely to be lower than that of the general population suffering from similar problems. Nevertheless, when using data obtained from controlled studies, it appears that avoidance is a prominent reason for dropping out of therapy for PTSD.

To specifically address the question of who drops out of therapy for PTSD, Bryant et al. (2007) evaluated a group of civilian trauma survivors who had been involved in vehicular accidents and nonsexual assaults. They randomly assigned participants to a series of CBT types of therapies, including those involving graded exposure, in vivo exposure, imaginal exposure, and cognitive restructuring. Approximately 25% of this motivated group dropped out of treatment before completion, and the authors identified two factors for dropping out. One was a tendency to engage in catastrophic thinking about their experience, and the other was a clear tendency toward avoidance:

> Participants who enter therapy with strong tendencies to avoid aversive events, not surprisingly, tend to avoid the demands of therapy by dropping out. . . . It is possible that treatment drop-out is most likely when someone catastrophises about treatment effects, and they then respond with avoidance. (Bryant et al., 2007, p. 15)

Imel, Laska, Jakupcak, and Simpson (2013) conducted a carefully controlled meta-analysis to analyze the possible causes of treatment dropout for those suffering from PTSD. The studies within the meta-analysis varied in terms of the degree to which the therapy entailed a focus on experienced traumatic events. So, for example, at one end of this spectrum would be *prolonged exposure (PE) therapy*, which requires the client to repeatedly confront the trauma. At the other end would be a therapy that minimally focuses on the traumatic event, such as *present-centered therapy* (PCT; Schnurr et al., 2003). PCT focuses on the nature of the symptoms of PTSD (i.e., psychoeducation), the development of effective coping strategies for day-to-day challenges that may result from PTSD, homework to monitor stressors, and the practice of new problem-solving strategies but little in the way of directly confronting PTSD-producing stimuli. Among the findings were that the degree to which the therapies focused on traumatic events did not affect the dropout rate. One important exception to those findings was that trauma-focused treatments resulted in a higher dropout rate than PCT, "a treatment originally designed as a control but now listed as a research-supported treatment for PTSD" ("Meta-Analysis of Dropout in Treatments for Posttraumatic Stress Disorder," 2016, p. 838). The authors concluded, "More research is needed comparing trauma-focused interventions to trauma-avoidant treatments such as PCT" ("Meta-Analysis of Dropout in Treatments for Posttraumatic Stress Disorder," 2016, p. 838). The results of the study clearly point to avoidance as being an important contributor to trauma treatment dropout.

In another study that examined treatment dropout—in this case, from trauma-focused cognitive behavior therapy (TF-CBT; Yasinski et al., 2018)—avoidance was again found to be the primarily contributor to dropout. The sample was diverse and included Medicaid-eligible youths (ages 7–17; $n = 108$) and their nonoffending caregivers ($n = 86$), who received TF-CBT through an effectiveness study in a community setting. The youths had experienced a variety of traumas, including sexual abuse, domestic violence, traumatic loss, accidents, and house fires. The children and caregivers displayed treatment dropout nearing 40%, and the results indicated that the trauma-focused nature of the treatment combined with a tendency to avoid dealing with trauma memories were the principal causes for treatment noncompletion.

The need to further explore treatments that do not focus on trauma memories, like the alternative therapies presented in this book, appears to be important in reducing potential treatment dropout. Recall that avoidance of trauma memories is one of the defining criteria of PTSD in the *DSM*. Thus, it would seem that therapies that deemphasize trauma recall would be more tolerable and likely to result in fewer dropouts than those that emphasize trauma recall. Although the Imel et al. (2013) study is not solid proof that avoidance of trauma memories is a significant factor in treatment dropout, the results of their study appear to strongly point in that direction. PCT not only resulted in lower treatment dropout but also turned out to be an effective treatment of PTSD. Many of the alternative therapies presented in this volume do not require that clients confront trauma memories, and like PCT, are likely to have lower dropout rates.

In another study, Garcia, Kelley, Rentz, and Lee (2011) examined dropout rates from CBT therapies among veterans the wars in Iraq and Afghanistan. They particularly focused on pretreatment predictors rather than the nature of the therapy itself. Using a PTSD symptom checklist, these researchers found that avoidance/numbing, hyperarousal, and reexperiencing were all highly associated with dropout from treatment. What this study and the aforementioned ones strongly suggest, although perhaps do not directly "prove," is that the extreme discomfort created by having to recall and reprocess unpleasant and unwanted memories of trauma may be significantly associated with treatment avoidance and dropout before treatment completion. Undoubtedly, clients drop out of treatment for PTSD for many reasons, but avoidance of unpleasant trauma memories appears to be a major factor. For this reason, alternatives to traditional CBT treatments that involve confronting trauma memories are needed. A somewhat typical case of treatment avoidance appears later in the chapter.

Costs of PTSD

It is estimated that 5% to 7% of Americans have PTSD at any given time, figures that translate into more than 15 million people. About 8% will develop the disorder in their lifetime. These numbers bespeak a huge psychological cost related to PTSD. Women are nearly twice as likely to develop PTSD than men, and younger people are more likely to develop the disorder following trauma experiences than older individuals (Motta, 2015).

These trauma experiences and the resultant PTSD typically lead to four symptom clusters. The first involves reliving the event through nightmares, painful and intrusive memories, or sudden rushes to heart thumping, fast breathing, and elevated blood pressure. Sweating, jitteriness, and fear follow. The second symptom cluster is "the big one": avoiding consciously or unconsciously any thoughts, feelings, images, sensations, or perceptions that remind the sufferer of the traumatic event. The reason this is referred to as "the big one" is that it is also the cluster that makes psychotherapy so difficult or, at times, impossible. If the sufferer is avoiding psychic pain at all costs and the therapist is urging the confrontation of this pain, then the client simply avoids the source of the problem: the therapist. Avoidance is the primary reason why traditional therapies fail. The third cluster of symptoms involves hyperarousal. The traumatized individual is on guard, wary, alert, and ready to enact survival behaviors they believe keep them safe. This often means they distance themselves from others, dampen feelings, and do not make commitments. Hyperarousal is the armor, the protective barrier that keeps threats of future attacks at bay. The fourth symptom cluster is a disturbance of cognition and mood. Those with PTSD have difficulty with memory and concentration. It is almost as if their preoccupation with the trauma interferes with all areas of cognitive functioning. This preoccupation eventuates in depressive and anxious mood states.

These responses to trauma are a heavy price to pay for the individual who lives a double life as a member of society and of a traumatized underworld of threat and fear of annihilation. It is a heavy price for society to pay, too. PTSD is staggeringly costly to treat. It is difficult to derive actual costs, but in 1 year, the Veterans Health Administration treated more than 100,000 cases of PTSD from the wars in Iraq and Afghanistan at a cost of more than $8,000 per person per year (Congressional Budget Office, 2012). So, the cost for these 100,000 cases was $800 million for 1 year. Because treatment usually continues for many years, the costs run into the billions of dollars. But the majority of veterans with PTSD did not seek treatment; they avoided it. Estimating the cost of treating more than 15 million cases for multiple years of treatment is both staggering and unimaginable.

Incidents That Produce PTSD

Although the cost estimates of treating PTSD come primarily from the Veterans Health Administration and are war related, these military cases actually represent a comparatively small percentage of incidents that produce PTSD. A number of other sources may put people at risk of developing the disorder, including survivors who may repeatedly face or have witnessed violent or life-threatening situations, such as war, school or workplace shootings, terrorist attacks, physical or sexual assault, rape, abuse, domestic violence, robbery, or critical illness. Survivors may be either children or adults who are the victims of verbal, sexual, or physical abuse, or were as children. In addition, survivors may have survived events that are part of everyday life, such as hurricanes, vehicular accidents, plane crashes, or other disasters, or the death of a close friend or family member. Professionals such as first responders who come to the aid of victims of trauma also are at risk of developing PTSD.

Up to this point, I have not discussed one category of traumatized individuals: those having close, personal contact with a traumatized individual. Thus, trauma can spread to family members and close friends, and even to mental health professionals who treat traumatized individuals. This form of trauma is referred to by terms such as *secondary trauma, vicarious trauma,* and *compassion fatigue.* An example of secondary trauma would be parents traumatized by learning their daughter was raped and experiencing her emotional devastation. Regrettably, trauma has a contagious aspect to it in addition to being a major problem in and of itself.

CASE EXAMPLE: AVOIDING ANXIETY-PROVOKING MEMORIES

Peter arrived at my office and told me a disturbing story that led to his PTSD of 30 years standing. He was tormented and wanted to share his story with me because I was a former soldier and would "get" him. He related that when he was young, he had been a door gunner in a helicopter in the same outfit I had been assigned to in Vietnam, the First Cavalry Division. Now an assistant principal in a neighboring school district, he related that for decades, he slept no more than 3 hours a night, that he has been plagued by nightmares, and in a throwback to his army days, he would get up every night to "patrol the perimeter" (i.e., he peeked through the windows of his house to make sure there were no intruders). The specific incident that was causing Peter so much grief occurred one day when his helicopter was making a combat assault, which involved landing in an area where soldiers had observed the enemy. Peter expected that he and the enemy would both be giving and taking gunfire. The shocking incident occurred when Peter, firing away in the open door of the helicopter with his M60 machine gun, saw himself shoot a child. He didn't mean to do so, but in a combat assault, everyone is shooting, and chaos abounds. This image of his cutting down a child was indeed horrific and had caused him torment for decades.

I felt fortunate to be in a position to help this deeply troubled man. Unfortunately, I was less knowledgeable about trauma treatment than I am now. I informed him that we would have to go over what happened in detail because the technique of "exposure" seemed to have good empirical backing for treating PTSD—or so I believed at the time. I further informed Peter that I would make every effort to not overwhelm him because recounting this episode could be difficult for him, so we would proceed at a slow, tolerable pace. Peter was thankful that he would finally be able to overcome his tormenting past. We agreed to meet the following Tuesday at 4:00 p.m., a time that worked for him. He seemed eager for the next session.

And then I got a bitter lesson about treating PTSD that troubles me to this day and is one of the motivations for writing about treatment alternatives. I never heard from Peter again. I've recalled this incident numerous times over the years, and the likely candidate for his disappearance was that he scared himself out of therapy. I called him a week after his missed appointment to find out what happened. All he would say is that telling me about his traumatic experiences made him feel even worse than before, and he therefore could not come back to therapy. I believe that his telling me the story of what happened brought long-suppressed agonizing images back to his full awareness. He must have vividly seen himself descending in that helicopter, firing his machine gun, and killing a child. This imagery would likely have caused horrific anxiety for him. The thought of having to recount this incident in future sessions was too much for Peter to take.

In the beginning, all looked well for the matchup involving me as the clinician and Peter as the client. We both had served in the army at about the same time in Vietnam and had been in the same unit. Who better to understand him? Unfortunately, I don't think I fully understood the power of the avoidance response in those early days, although maybe I should have. Peter taught me an important lesson, and I pray that he eventually found peace. The avoidance response is the bane of clinicians who treat PTSD.

The need for therapies that do not evoke the strong, semireflexive avoidance response should be clear from this case example. Although traditional therapies may work for traumatized individuals who endure them, most will be unable to deal with the therapeutic process. What is called for are forms of intervention that clients can tolerate more easily and perhaps a pace that is far slower than what one often encounters. The therapist, eager to affect a "cure," often pushes the client at a pace they cannot tolerate. I am reminded of a stance taken in trauma therapist Peter Levine's (2010) book, *In an Unspoken Voice: How the Body Releases Trauma and Restores Goodness*, which is that in treating trauma, you can never go too slowly. When one moves too quickly, clients simply become overwhelmed and flee the therapeutic situation, and they frequently do not return. As a psychological practitioner and director of a university-based trauma clinic, I've seen a number of clients quit therapy after the first session during which they had described their traumatic experience, even if the clinician had said nearly nothing. In those cases, the clients had scared themselves out of therapy regardless of how slowly the clinician had been willing to move. By recounting their trauma, they experienced so much anxiety, they avoided future sessions that they believed would be similarly anxiety provoking.

This book cannot cover all alternatives to traditional psychotherapies that might be of value in treating PTSD or components of PTSD and trauma reactions, such as anxiety, depression, dissociation, and hypervigilance, even though hundreds of approaches claim to be effective in treating some or all of these components. It would be impossible to cover all possible therapeutic approaches. So, in this volume, I have selected approaches that have some level of compelling empirical support, and I have done so with the full realization that effective approaches may exist for which no empirical support is available.

OVERVIEW OF PTSD

Although the negative impact of traumatic experiences has been recognized throughout recorded history, the term *posttraumatic stress disorder* was identified only recently. There have been disagreements over its characteristics, the degree to which it alters human functioning, and how it should be treated. What follows is an overview of its history and treatment.

Brief History of PTSD

PTSD is a disorder that results when a person has witnessed or experienced life-threatening events or terrifying situations (Motta, 2013). For centuries, reactions to traumatic events "have been alluded to as far back as Homer's 'Iliad' and noted in literary heroes and heroines [who suffered intrusive recollections and nightmares] including Shakespeare's *Henry IV* (Trimble, 1985)" (Motta, 2015, p. 72). Other documented examples of PTSD are the 1666 writings of Samuel Pepys, who described having trouble sleeping and experiencing night terrors after living through the Great Fire of London (Daly, 1983). Stories from the Civil War by those who had not sustained physical injuries suggest such trauma reactions as a rapidly beating heart, irritability, and increased arousal. American physician Jacob Méndes Da Costa described those reactions, which came to be called Da Costa's syndrome (Clark, 1903). Some referred to the condition as irritable heart syndrome or Soldier's irritable heart, which is now seen as having more of an emotional than physiological etiology (Motta, 2015). Similar emotional responses known as railway spine resulted from accidents during the early days of railway development; the belief was that the reactions to that trauma were neurologically based (Trimble, 1981). The more contemporary terms such as *shell shock* and *rape trauma syndrome* seem to describe PTSD symptoms (Motta, 2015).

    PTSD first entered the diagnostic nomenclature with the publication of the third edition of the *DSM* (third ed. [*DSM–III*]; American Psychiatric Association, 1980), and the psychological casualties of the Vietnam War were one of the primary reasons for its inclusion in that text. The *DSM–III* "alluded to traumatic events that were 'beyond the range of normal human experience'" (Motta, 2013, p. 6). The *DSM–III* eventually dropped that criterion when evidence surfaced showing that common stressors like life-threatening illnesses, child neglect and abuse, and vehicular accidents could also produce the disorder (Motta, 2013).

Review of PTSD Symptoms

Those interested in learning about PTSD will often go to the *DSM*, where the disorder is defined primarily by its symptoms, including mood difficulties, problems of concentration and memory, the tendency to startle easily, nightmares, unwanted vivid recollections of traumatic events, and hyperarousal. What is lacking in this description of PTSD is what this disorder does to one's sense of self and one's perception of the environment. The person suffering from PTSD often sees themselves differently than they did before they were traumatized. This new self is generally a more dehumanized version of the former self such that one may now view themselves as more remote, more suspicious, and wearier. Trauma has animalized them; whereas previously they may have felt secure, they now feel that the environment has the potential to harm them. Those with PTSD not only feel uncomfortable in their own skin but also distrust their surroundings (Motta, 2013).

People who encounter traumatic events typically do not develop PTSD. According to Breslau (2009), approximately 7% of traumatized individuals develop the group of symptoms that eventuate in a diagnosis of PTSD. In general, as the traumatic stressors increase so does the probability of being diagnosed with PTSD. Combatants in the Vietnam War had rates of PTSD of approximately 15%, whereas children and adolescents traumatized by the terrorism of the Khmer Rouge in Cambodia had rates nearing 100% (Motta, 2013). These same children, 3 years later, showed rates of 50% (Kinzie, Sack, Angell, Clarke, & Ben, 1989). Foster care children who have been sexually abused have been found to have PTSD rates nearing 70% (Dubner & Motta, 1999), whereas those who were in foster care because of physical abuse had rates of approximately 40%. In general, females are more likely to develop PTSD than males, children are more vulnerable to having the disorder than those who are older, and those who may have had emotional adjustment difficulties before being traumatized are more likely to develop PTSD than those who were previously well adjusted (Motta, 2013). Anyone who is unfortunate enough to have been diagnosed with PTSD will experience a life that has been negatively altered in multiple ways, and these negative alterations can often continue for many years.

Diagnostic Criteria for PTSD

It is most common to describe the symptoms of PTSD in a recipelike fashion by delineating specific symptoms. According to the *DSM–5* (American Psychiatric Association, 2013), following exposure to threatened or actual death, sexual violence, serious injury, or similarly frightening experience, many individuals develop characteristic symptoms:

- They may experience intrusive symptoms, such as recurrent, involuntary distressing memories and dreams. These unwanted experiences could be so intense they precipitate dissociative reactions that, in the extreme, cause a complete loss of awareness of present surroundings.

- Individuals may persistently avoid stimuli linked to traumatic event. As indicated earlier, this avoidance, although often conscious, can also occur below the level of consciousness, thus presenting one of the major difficulties in treating PTSD.

- Negative alterations in cognition and mood may occur. Cognitive alterations can be reflected in statements or thoughts like "I'm bad" or, "You can't trust anyone." Mood alterations can include the inability to experience pleasure; detachment or estrangement from others; an inability to love; or feelings of fear, anger, guilt, depression.

- Individuals may experience marked alterations in arousal and reactivity that can manifest as irritability and angry outbursts, exaggerated startle responses, hypervigilance, sleep problems, and problems of concentration.

- For a diagnosis of PTSD, the preceding symptoms must last at least 1 month and cause clinically significant distress. It is not uncommon, though, for PTSD to last a lifetime. World War II veterans bordering on 90 years of age have reported bouts of sleeplessness, startle responses, and unwanted intrusive imagery all related to their war experiences. I left Vietnam more than 4 decades ago and find that I still startle with fear on hearing noises like fireworks or anything that sounds like gunfire. Truth be told, I left the country every Fourth of July for 10 years after returning from the war to avoid those life-threatening (to me) sounds.

Another facet of PTSD, which is of central importance and is often not emphasized in the *DSM*, is the alteration of one's sense of self and view of one's environment. People who have been traumatized often report they are not the same person they used to be and they no longer see the environment as they used to. Those who are traumatized have been known to view themselves as older, more negative, more suspicious, and perhaps lacking in humanity. They have a tendency to see the environment as threatening and unwelcoming. One's basic assumptions about the world are shaken and then called into question. They may no longer hold assumptions such as "honesty is the best policy," "hard work leads to success," "we are all caring human beings" as strongly as before. The experience of trauma is often so shocking and devastating that it produces a realignment of oneself with one's environment. One's basic assumptions of their environment seem to no longer be valid (McCann & Pearlman, 1990). So, PTSD is more than a recipe of symptoms; it is also an alteration of one's self-view and view of the environment, and this alteration can sometimes last a lifetime. It would not be farfetched to say that PTSD can transform an individual from a human being into a frightened, weary animal—sometimes for life.

Developmental Trauma and Complex PTSD

Most of the literature and research on PTSD deals with disruptive events, such as war, rape, sexual assault, vehicular accidents, and natural disasters, that appear to occupy a limited and difficult time in people's lives. Another type of traumatization involves stressors that are experienced over longer periods and include such events as experiencing prolonged physical, sexual, or emotional abuse; neglect in childhood; or chronic intimate partner violence; or being kidnapped, held hostage, forced into becoming a member of a religious cult, or taken as a prisoner of war. Situations involving being captive or trapped for extended periods can lead to this disorder. *Complex PTSD* (C-PTSD), a term that appears to have been coined by Judith Herman (1992), is often associated with developmental traumas, such as those that begin in childhood and continue for long periods, but can apply to any long-running trauma experience. These forms of trauma are referred to as DESNOS (disorders of extreme stress not otherwise specified in the *DSM*) or as C-PTSD in the *International Classification of Diseases for Mortality and Morbidity Statistics, 11th Revision* (World Health Organization, 2018), or as developmental trauma disorder (van der Kolk, 2005). Some have debated whether C-PTSD is simply a variant of PTSD, but research suggests it does have distinct differences from PTSD and borderline personality disorder (BPD); BPD is associated with disrupted childhood upbringing.

A study conducted by Cloitre, Garvert, Weiss, Carlson, and Bryant (2014) involving 280 women examined differences between C-PTSD, PTSD, and BPD. The study found that those with C-PTSD showed high levels of PTSD symptoms in addition to high levels of disorganization involving affect regulation. Explosions of anger are not uncommon in C-PTSD. In contrast, those with PTSD had low levels of disturbance in self-regulation of affect. Those with C-PTSD had a generally negative view of relationships, a deeply negative sense of self, and a tendency toward self-isolation. Those in the BPD group showed varying levels of engagement and trust of others, and also variations in self-concept in contrast to the persistently negative self-concept seen in C-PTSD. From this study, it would seem that C-PTSD often has a more pervasive negative impact than does PTSD. With PTSD, one might be able to conceive of their trauma as an isolated, yet highly troubling event. In C-PTSD, the trauma seems to define the self in a more pervasive and enduring negative way.

According to some authors (e.g., Cloitre et al., 2009), a central defining characteristic of C-PTSD is that it is "driven by the interpersonal nature of most of the traumas . . ." (p. 8). C-PTSD often emerges from a history of sustained disruption of early childhood attachments. These attachments are frequently characterized by abuse and maltreatment from which there is little possibility of escape and that eventuate in intense fear and feelings of unpredictability and dread. The intensely insecure attachments that result in C-PTSD create particular difficulties for the treating clinician.

When beginning treatment with a child, the first issue for the clinician is to address and identify any ongoing threats to the safety of that child, and to also ensure safety and stability. The focus of treatment then involves developing an emotional bridge that emphasizes trust, predictability, and security. This phase of treatment cannot be rushed and can take a number of months before a safe and secure relationship develops. The emphasis of treatment at this early stage should also be emotion regulation and take a somewhat pragmatic approach to dealing with interpersonal problems and finding effective ways of handling life's frustrations. Only after taking these steps should the clinician begin—with the client's consent—to move toward a recall and reprocessing of the traumatic event or events. A hopeful outcome of this process is the development of a perspective in which the trauma or traumas do not define the individual but rather are seen as a part of the whole person. With treatment, the client hopefully views the traumas as experiences that have taken place in one's life but no longer take the role of the only experiences or the most important experiences. At all points in treatment, the clinician should emphasize safety. It takes considerable courage on a child or adult client's part to begin to trust. It also requires a good deal of patience and caring on the part of the clinician to foster these feelings of safety and security. Treating PTSD requires that clinicians take great care to not overwhelm the client. This careful approach is especially called for in treating C-PTSD.

Disasters and PTSD

The available research (e.g., Boscarino, Adams, Figley, Galea, & Foa, 2006) appears to point to trauma experiences of human design, such as muggings, assaults, abuse, and rapes, as having a more negative and enduring emotional impact on individuals than those involving disasters of various kinds. Some have suggested that clients may perceive the experiences of human design as more personal and intentional than those involving disasters, and that perception adds to the experienced distress. This research is particularly relevant to C-PTSD, which is of an intensely personal and enduring nature. Research on remission rates (e.g., Morina, Wicherts, Lobbrecht, & Priebe, 2014) show that PTSD resulting from natural disaster has the highest remission rate—after 10 months—of 60% compared with the lowest of 31% for those who have experienced a physical disease. Personal attacks of various kinds have remission rates somewhere between these two. Morina et al. (2014) suggested that the reason for the lower remission rate among those who have experienced physical illness may be that these persons carry the illness that caused PTSD; thus, they may be constantly reminded of this stressor while also being less able to physically cope with it. From earlier discussion in this chapter, it is apparent that a large number of variables are associated with the development of PTSD, including age, gender, socioeconomic status, premorbid adjustment, social support, type of trauma, perceived personal nature of the trauma, and duration of trauma.

Within the field of disasters and PTSD are subdivisions of study, including human-created disasters, such as terrorist attacks in New York and many other areas across the globe; technological and accidental disasters, such as Chernobyl or the Exxon Valdez oil spill; natural disasters, such as earthquakes, cyclones, tsunamis, hurricanes, and tornados; and those that appear to combine human-created and natural disasters, such as intentionally initiated forest fires (Neria, Nandi, & Galea, 2008). Other subdivisions of study include traumas resulting when individuals, for example, first responders, observe people in a disaster either in person or through the media. To complicate matters further, traumas can arise from close involvement with someone who has been traumatized because of a disaster, personal attack, or some form of complex traumatization (McCann & Pearlman, 1990; Motta, 2008).

The literature on what happens after a disaster points to consistent estimates of how disasters affect one's development of PTSD (Neria et al., 2008). According to Neria et al. (2008),

> the prevalence of PTSD among direct victims of disasters ranges between 30% and 40%; the range of PTSD prevalence among rescue workers is lower, ranging between 10% and 20%; while the range in the general population is lowest and expected to be between 5% and 10%. (p. 5)

Furthermore, it appears that across studies, the most consistent determinant of the risk of PTSD is the severity of the exposure to the event. Of particular importance are the immediate risk to life, how severely property was destroyed, the extent of physical injuries, and how often fatalities occurred (Neria et al., 2008). Responses to trauma, regardless of type, appear to follow a consistent pattern that is highlighted in various iterations of the *DSM*. The alterations of one's reactions to their environment, including distrust, anxiety, and altered sense of self, following a traumatic experience are fairly consistent regardless of the nature of the trauma experience. The standard of treatment for PTSD resulting from disasters involves a reprocessing of the disaster experiences through CBT approaches. Well-controlled studies of alternative therapies for disasters that involve random assignment and control are virtually nonexistent, but there is no reason to believe that alternative approaches would not be of value in treating this form of trauma.

CRITICAL VALUE OF THE THERAPEUTIC RELATIONSHIP

A common saying is that the relationship between the therapist and the client is the sine qua non of psychotherapy. This Latin term is translated as "without which nothing," meaning that the therapeutic relationship is of critical importance in psychotherapy and that without this essential element, little progress is likely to take place. Although this adage may be true for the treatment of most psychological problems, it is particularly important in treating PTSD because traumatized children, adolescents, and adults commonly have problems with trust and have particular difficulty with trusting relationships. PTSD sufferers have often been hurt within the context of a relationship and therefore do not readily trust. It is essential that the PTSD sufferer be convinced that his or her therapist "gets" them and will make every effort to provide help without overwhelming them. Should the client begin to feel overwhelmed by having to confront extremely anxiety-provoking material, they frequently will quit therapy and will avoid. For this reason, the clinician should emphasize developing a caring and trusting relationship before they and the client wade into the frightening waters of PTSD-causing experiences.

A study that assessed the value of the therapeutic alliance in successful completion of treatment for PTSD for a variety of traumas in an adult sample (Keller, Zoellner, & Feeny, 2010) found that the quality of the therapeutic alliance is associated with better treatment engagement, better adherence, and less dropout across a range of treatments and disorders. The authors concluded that the alliance was critical for treatment completion and success. What is surprising is that this was the case even for a treatment emphasizing PE and also involving sample members who had experienced child sexual abuse. Often those experiencing such abuse are particularly resistant to treatment, especially when it involves being continually exposed to traumatic material. A history of sexual abuse was not a predictor of treatment engagement and adherence, whereas the alliance between therapist and client was.

One of the problems frequently seen in the psychotherapy literature is an overemphasis on techniques of therapy with comparatively less attention to the therapeutic relationship. Where PTSD is concerned, this emphasis on techniques highlights the value of CBT types of treatment. It is almost as if there is a prevailing view that if therapists use the most effective techniques, we will obtain the most "cures." A good deal of the research literature is a comparison of one treatment to another and often uses random assignment and placebo controls with little attention to the relationship in therapy. All of this has a scientific and valid ring to it, but it is important to recall that such studies frequently involve highly motivated volunteers who willingly participate in such randomly controlled trials. The findings may be relevant only to participants who are similarly motivated and not to the general population who are often treatment avoidant. The emphasis on the comparison of various techniques camouflages or overshadows the critical value of the therapeutic relationship. It appears that what is actually resulting in significant improvement in the treatment of PTSD is a combination of effective treatment within a context of a trusting, mutually respectful and caring relationship, but many studies often treat the relationship as a stepchild.

Wampold et al. (2010) carefully reviewed a series of meta-analyses regarding what actually works in the treatment of PTSD. These meta-analyses examined an array of bona fide treatments, some of which claimed to specifically focus on the trauma during therapy, some of which did not, and some of which altered between a focus on trauma and one on what might be referred to as psychoeducation regarding the nature of trauma and its impact on individuals. A large number of variables were identified as important in trauma treatment, but Wampold et al. did not find any one particular type of therapy to be more effective than others in the overall treatment of PTSD. What these authors did find as important issues were elements such as ensuring safety of the client; developing a trusting, respectful relationship between clinician and client; agreeing on the goals of therapy and the tasks to be undertaken; creating an opportunity for the client to talk about their trauma; cultivating a sense of self-efficacy and hope; providing psychoeducation about PTSD; teaching the client coping and survival skills in addition to helping them identify their strengths; assisting clients to learn how to avoid revictimization; exposing the client to the trauma (although therapies that avoided exposure were also effective); taking a look at the behavioral chain of events; and helping the client make sense of their experience of trauma and reaction to it (Wampold et al., 2010). These authors would likely agree that fitting a particular treatment strategy to a particular client who has unique strengths and weaknesses and who has experienced specific forms of trauma is far more important than seeking out a particular therapy based on its theoretical rationale or its representation of a unique school of therapy.

TRADITIONAL TREATMENTS FOR PTSD

The definition of what is a traditional versus nontraditional treatment of PTSD is somewhat arbitrary. Although psychoanalysis was once a traditional and gold standard of therapy, CBT and PE are now the accepted approaches and, for many, the traditional and most effective way of treating trauma. "The treatment of choice for PTSD . . . is exposure based cognitive therapy" (Preston, O'Neal, & Talaga, 2002, p. 137). For our purposes, I define *traditional treatment* as that family of methods claiming to have acquired the most empirical support for their efficacy over the years. All such "claims" have their detractors. Although the current view is that CBT interventions have the most empirical support, some have expressed doubt over how much support has actually been demonstrated. For example, many empirical studies of CBT have compared this intervention to no-treatment controls or treatment as usual. CBT naysayers would assert that just about any treatment would show itself to be better than no treatment. The naysayers might also state that rather than compare CBT with treatment as usual, why not compare it with a bona fide intervention, such as those therapies that emphasize the value of the therapeutic relationship (Wampold, 2015)?

Another line of critique of CBT is that it is often carried out by those who are adherents of the procedure and that some form of experimenter bias may be operating (Leichsenring & Steinert, 2017). Practitioners and researchers, including me, might argue that the focus on cognitions in CBT misses the mark. The problems encountered with PTSD are not dysfunctional thoughts but rather extreme and problematic emotions, primarily anxiety, that are activated almost reflexively by a multitude of stimuli in the current environment. PTSD does not typically involve a cortically based thinking dysfunction; rather, it is a subcortical, reflexive fear. Despite these concerns, CBT has undergone many empirical investigations, and although it may lack wholehearted support, it is considered by many to be the traditional and accepted treatment of PTSD. I intentionally use the term *considered* here because CBT has not been extensively tested and accepted as a form of PTSD treatment that is superior to other forms of treatment. It is simply a well-tested form of treatment for many forms of emotional dysfunction, such as anxiety and depression.

With its focus on correcting dysfunctional cognitions or making PTSD sufferers more rational, CBT seems to miss the mark. PTSD is far less about one's illogical thoughts and much more about one's extreme and seemingly reflexive emotional reactivity. Here's a personal example. For many years after my return home from the Vietnam War, the Fourth of July was a real problem for me. I would be on the verge of panic when the "explosions" from the fireworks began and would hide in the basement next to the furnace.

While there, I asked myself questions as a CBT therapist might do: "Do you know you are safe and that this is just a celebratory holiday?"

"Yes," I answered myself.

"Are you sure you are safe—even 100% sure?"

"Yes" was again the answer.

"Are you certain you will not be hurt?"

"Yes, I'm certain."

I was convinced that I was in no danger and that I was below ground level and was completely and unquestionably safe. In other words, my thoughts or cognitions were perfectly rational. CBT with its emphasis on correcting irrational thoughts would have been of no help to me. Despite my rational thinking, I was having a panic attack. It should be clear from this example that PTSD and trauma reactions are far less about irrational or dysfunctional thoughts and far more about conditioned emotional reactions that have almost nothing to do with thinking. For many, but perhaps not all of those with PTSD, cognitively based therapeutic interventions are of little value.

Many practitioners consider trauma-focused therapies like CBT, cognitive processing therapy (CPT), and TF-CBT as widely accepted first-line treatment for PTSD. Bradley et al. (2005) conducted a meta-analysis of these techniques in treating PTSD and found them to be equally effective, having a clinical improvement level of 44%. A nonexhaustive selection of these "traditional" CBT therapies include the following.

Rational Emotive Therapy and Rational Emotive Behavior Therapy

Rational emotive therapy (RET; Ellis, 1975) was one of the first approaches from which the newer "third wave" therapies, such as acceptance and commitment therapy (ACT; Hayes, Strosahl, & Wilson, 2016) and dialectical behavior therapy (DBT; Linehan, 1993), evolved. RET maintains that much of human suffering and self-denigration arises from irrational thoughts such as, "I must be competent in all things I do," "I must be loved and approved of by everyone," and "It would be awful if I were rejected." These thoughts are seen as lacking in objective reality and ultimately lead to feelings of negativity and worthlessness. The underlying model on which treatment for PTSD is based is the *ABC model* (Ellis, 1994): *A*, an activating event or disturbing experience, is often followed by *B*, beliefs that may be irrational like those described previously, and these beliefs lead to *C*, emotional "consequences" and a negative self-view. The initial development of RET involved a primary focus on irrational thoughts, and therapy entailed a depropagandizing or disabusing the client of these irrational beliefs through cognitive disputation of them. Much of RET involved having the client challenge the irrationality of their thinking.

Rational emotive behavior therapy (Ellis, 1975) incorporated a behavioral component whereby clients would not only challenge their dysfunctional thinking but also engage in behaviors that brought about positive change. Thus, rational emotive behavior therapy often incorporated assertiveness training exercises and *shame attacks* in which the client would publicly engage in behaviors that would draw unwanted attention to themselves, such as loudly announcing the time to patrons of a crowded restaurant. The purpose of this behavioral component was to practice adaptive behavior and to see that even the disapproval of others for outlandish behavioral displays as in shame attacks was endurable rather than terrible or catastrophic.

Acceptance and Commitment Therapy

The objective of ACT (Hayes et al., 2016) is not to eliminate unwanted and unacceptable feelings but rather to be present with whatever life brings and to move toward more valued adaptive behavior. To some extent, this form of therapy involves an acceptance of what is rather than an attempt to neutralize unpleasant thoughts and feelings and then to move toward what matters most to the individual. ACT and other CBT approaches incorporate mindfulness practices, which are arguably not within the realm of CBT, which emphasizes altering dysfunctional cognitions and developing adaptive behaviors. Perhaps that is the rationale for the designation of "third wave" of ACT-like therapies (i.e., an emphasis on meditative and contemplative practices reflective of eastern traditions).

Dialectal Behavior Therapy

Central to DBT (Linehan, 1993) is the acceptance of change, emotion regulation, and distress tolerance. In treating clients using DBT, the therapist aims to be the client's partner rather than adversary ("Dialectical Behavior Therapy," n.d.). The therapist takes the position of encouraging the client to accept their dysfunctional behaviors as a response to an invalidating upbringing or circumstances. At the same time, they work with the client to see that these behaviors are maladaptive and that, for the client's benefit, adaptive behaviors are to be developed. Thus, the client is committing to acceptance and change by appreciating the dialectics principle, which is thesis plus antithesis leads to synthesis, and is using an array of skills for the purpose of developing emotional self-regulation (Fatwa, n.d.). The dialectic in this case involves an acceptance and validation of the way one is while also accepting the importance of adaptive change.

Eastern traditions, such as mindfulness meditation, are also incorporated into DBT so that one can learn to accept oneself and one's present situation nonjudgmentally. DBT is the standard treatment for clients with BPD (Linehan, 1993), and many of these clients have suffered from traumatic experiences and PTSD. DBT includes four modules: mindfulness, distress tolerance, emotion regulation, and interpersonal effectiveness. Mindfulness involves observing, describing, and participating nonjudgmentally in moment-to-moment experience and thus borrows from the Buddhist tradition. Distress tolerance involves accepting, rather than becoming overwhelmed by, negative situations and their effects. One is taught to accept without evaluating oneself and the current situation ("Dialectical Behavior Therapy," n.d.). Thus, the first two modules, mindfulness and distress tolerance, appear to have a basis in Eastern traditions of observation and acceptance, while the other two, emotion regulation and interpersonal effectiveness, rely more so on Western cognitive and behavioral approaches to treatment.

Prolonged Exposure

Based in emotional processing theory, PE hypothesizes that PTSD symptoms result from

> cognitive and behavioral avoidance of trauma-related thoughts, reminders, activities and situations [e.g., Foa et al., 2007; Foa & Kozak, 1986]. PE helps the client interrupt and reverse this process by blocking cognitive and behavioral avoidance, introducing corrective information, and facilitating organization and processing of the trauma memory and associated thoughts and beliefs. (Center for Deployment Psychology, n.d., para. 2)

The therapist achieves this process through *in vivo*, that is, in life or real-life, and *imaginal exposure*, that is, using one's imagination to redevelop trauma scenarios.

The focus of PE is to move from habitually avoiding unwanted thoughts and feelings to confronting them. Exhorting the client to deal directly with the thoughts, feelings, and memories, and other sensations and perceptions associated with the traumatic experience is one of the therapeutic goals. The therapist frequently records sessions and instructs the client to listen to the recordings at home. The U.S. Department of Veterans Affairs (VA) often uses PE for combatants traumatized by the horrors of war. Clinicians may ask clients to listen to the sounds of combat or view videos of combat situations, or to don virtual reality (VR) equipment to confront, as nearly as possible, the stimuli that precipitated PTSD. VA claims the approach to be successful in treating PTSD; however, what it doesn't report is that the majority of individuals who attempt the PE process quit because of the anxiety it evokes, and many report a worsening of symptoms (Morris, 2015). A few years ago, a colleague of mine who was enamored with VR equipment asked me to don the headgear and view a Vietnam combat scene. I lasted all of 3 seconds. The intense and visceral anxiety that the VR-based war scene evoked in me is difficult to describe. So much for my willingness to endure PE, VR, or any similar "treatment."

At this juncture, one must ask, What is the value of a therapeutic approach that is so difficult to endure that the majority will not tolerate it? The idea behind PE is that individuals will habituate to the stimuli associated with PTSD by repeated exposure to these stimuli. That position may be accurate but is akin to taking a child who is fearful of the water and throwing them in from a boat, and then doing so repeatedly. PE is a form of treatment that is difficult to tolerate but has a chance of neutralizing the fear of water, or trauma, for those willing and able to cope with it.

A far more client-friendly approach, which clinicians often use in the university-based trauma clinic that I direct, is a slow, graded form of exposure that involves simple discussion of one's trauma when and if the client is ready for such a discussion. The client dictates the pace of the discussion with gentle encouragement from the therapist. Treating a fear by way of prolonged and intensive exposure to the fear, and the consequent aversion to such approaches, is why alternatives to traditional interventions have a place in therapists' treatment arsenal. To repeat: "Alternative" therapies have come into existence because many of the traditional approaches, although potentially effective in improving the lives of PTSD sufferers, are so difficult to endure that clients avoid them altogether. The sad fact is that the majority of those who suffer from PTSD do not pursue psychotherapy because they see it as traumatizing. If this has a paradoxical ring to it, it should.

Cognitive Processing Therapy

Manualized forms of CBT are also common and have been used with adults, adolescents, and children. One such manualized form of CBT is CPT, developed initially for rape victims and now used in treating veterans with PTSD (Resick, 2001). Four essential elements of CPT are

- educating the client about the specifics of PTSD and why treatment might help,
- informing the client about their thoughts and feelings,
- helping the client challenge their dysfunctional thoughts, and

- helping the client recognize changes in their beliefs that happened after going through treatment.

A typical 12-session run of CPT has shown to be effective with veterans and others with PTSD if they are able to stay with the treatment and not quit. An initial session might involve psychoeducation, teaching the client about the nature of PTSD and CPT procedures. The two sessions that follow involve writing and reading about the traumatic event and why the client believed it happened. The clinician then tries to identify problematic beliefs about the traumatic event and determine how they have affected the client's perspectives and feelings (Motta, 2013). So, for example, the therapist might target the perceived ubiquity of these events and perceived self-blame for the events. They establish a link as to how these often incorrect beliefs can result in emotional distress (e.g., "So, Mary, can you see how blaming yourself leads to feelings of low self-worth and emotional pain?"). The therapist dedicates further sessions to helping the client learn how to challenge false beliefs. In remaining sessions, the client may use a variety of tools, such as logs or drawings, to challenge overgeneralizations in thinking such as, "You can't trust anyone," or, "I'm a bad person because of what happened." The clinician then teaches the client more adaptive ways of perceiving their environments (Alvarez et al., 2011). CPT heavily emphasizes the cognitive elements of CBT. The active challenging of one's beliefs and the subsequent development of adaptive behavioral strategies encompass behavioral methods commonly seen in CBT.

Limitations of This Overview

The preceding material on traditional interventions is in no way meant to be an exhaustive list. There is no agreed on compendium of CBT therapies. A partial listing of CBT therapies included in the book *Effective Treatments for PTSD* (Foa, Keane, & Friedman, 2000) includes exposure therapy, systematic desensitization, stress inoculation training, CPT, cognitive therapy, assertiveness training, biofeedback, and relaxation training. Some of these approaches are far more cognitive than behavioral and others, the reverse.

WHAT IS AN EFFECTIVE TREATMENT OF PTSD?

At first glance, the answer to this question should be obvious. It would seem that any approach that reduces the symptoms of PTSD under well-controlled experimental conditions would be considered to be an effective treatment. Before getting involved with definitions of what constitutes an effective treatment, we must ask ourselves, How effective is a treatment that causes its recipients to avoid it? Many of the cognitive and behavioral treatments have empirical evidence for their effectiveness in controlled experimental studies, but client aversion to these treatments in the real world is why they seek alternative therapies. Another problem in discussing treatment effectiveness is this question: From whose perspective are we discussing improvement? The therapist or researcher might consider a treatment effective if the client no longer withdraws from social interaction, no longer avoids situations they previously did, now shows improvements on standardized measures of PTSD, and perhaps shows reductions on scales measuring anxiety and depression. The PTSD sufferer might not care whether they improved on standardized measures or whether they no longer avoid situations that reminded them of their trauma. The sufferer might report that simply being happier and more hopeful are indications of improvement. Although the therapist or researcher might also value these improvements, they are difficult to measure and may not be considered indicators of "real" improvement. The point here is that what constitutes "improvement" might come down to a matter of definition, and clients and therapists may have different definitions.

This issue of who is being asked to evaluate the effectiveness of a treatment is not an academic question. It is of central importance in the therapy evaluation process. A number of years ago, a colleague and I (Motta & Lynch, 1990) conducted a study in which we used specific behavioral interventions with children, such as assertiveness training, token economies, and social skills training, to improve academic effort, increase adaptive behavior, and improve social functioning. Our results were positive and encouraging. When the therapists were asked what, in their view, resulted in positive changes in the children, they usually credited the specific therapeutic techniques they used. When parents were asked why the children improved, they usually pointed to the personal qualities of the therapist, such as empathic responding to the child's concerns and the therapists' befriending of the child. Also, in general, therapists saw greater degrees of positive change in the children than did parents, although both saw improvement as having occurred. So not only did the parents of the children rate the magnitude of change differently from that of the therapists, they also attributed the observed changes to different causes than did the therapists. So, who is right here? The available research shows that specific interventions and a caring relationship with a therapist both have therapeutic value, so perhaps everyone was right. Clearly, evaluating therapeutic effectiveness is no simple matter.

Meta-analytic studies that combine the results of numerous investigations point to the therapeutic relationship or alliance as the crucial variable underlying therapeutic change (Wampold, 2015), and yet theorists, dating even farther back than Sigmund Freud, have adamantly asserted that it is techniques of therapy that produce change in clients. Complicating matters still further, it is possible that therapeutic technique and the relationship are not so separable. After all, a caring therapist chooses techniques or approaches they believe will be most beneficial to the client.

A treatment issue sometimes seen in the literature is the distinction between treatment effectiveness and efficacy. *Effectiveness* often refers to the degree to which one can use the treatment with large numbers of people. Does the average PTSD sufferer benefit from the treatment? If so, the treatment is effective. The term *efficacy* is frequently used to describe the outcome of research studies; it refers to how a select group of participants receiving a specific intervention improved on standardized measures (i.e., instruments that are reliable and valid). Ideally, treatments should be both effective and efficacious, that is, the general population that suffers from PTSD accepts treatments, and these people show significant improvement on standardized measures. That may be the ideal, but it is not what is commonly seen. What is more often seen is that a select group of participants with specific definable characteristics tolerated a clearly specified treatment and completed the standardized measures. If they showed improvement on the standardized measures, then the treatment being researched would be considered efficacious, but not necessarily effective, because only a select group of individuals with specific characteristics were involved in the study. The general population of PTSD sufferers may have a whole amalgam of characteristics, not just those that would allow them to participate in a specific, highly controlled study using specific techniques for a specific period. Those not involved in a research study may have a variety of traumas, may be of varying ages and educations, and may have varied levels of discipline and psychological sophistication, but would not qualify to participate in the specific study. Thus, the question arises: Would the treatment efficacy demonstrated in a study having specific types of participants and using specific techniques or given amounts of time work in the general population? In other words, efficacy derived from a specific study using specific procedures may not be effective in that the results have not been shown to be broadly applicable.

SUMMARY

The preceding material on what constitutes an effective treatment is relevant to how we are to evaluate alternative therapies for PTSD. If we adhere to a standard of only accepting treatments for which there is demonstrated empirical support, then we are looking at the CBTs and PE interventions, and to a lesser, although acceptable extent, eye-movement desensitization and reprocessing (EMDR), which involves making alternating eye movements while holding elements of traumatic stimuli in awareness. Like CBT interventions, EMDR, which I cover in Chapter 2, has been granted the imprimatur of an empirically supported treatment but has not found wide acceptance among traditional CBT advocates or in the academic community because it does not fit handily into the learning theory model on which CBT is based. If the therapeutic community opens the field of investigation to interventions that do not have the level of empirical support that CBT has, then we are examining a group of interventions that are accepted and sought by a wide range of PTSD sufferers, and are also setting out to examine the utility of such interventions as yoga, mindfulness, acupuncture, and movement therapies.

The plan for this book is to start with a review of EMDR because therapists often view it as straddling the border between empirically supported treatments and alternative treatments. After a period of outright skepticism and rejection by the therapeutic community when EMDR first appeared, owing to its unorthodox methodology (i.e., it does not fitting into the orthodox learning theory paradigm enjoyed by traditional CBT approaches, and it emphasizes eye movements), it has now gained some degree of (grudging) support from the American Psychological Association, the VA, the World Health Organization, and others. Its difficulty in fitting into a traditional learning theory framework has resulted in many traditionalists and academics' seeing it as a pseudotherapy and therefore occupies a place somewhere on the border between traditional and alternative approaches.

2

Eye-Movement Desensitization and Reprocessing for PTSD

This chapter describes how eye-movement desensitization and reprocessing (EMDR) was developed as a treatment for trauma and how it is done. It also addresses the reluctance of the academic community to accept EMDR even though the American Psychological Association (APA Presidential Task Force on Evidence-Based Practice, 2006) has accepted EMDR as an empirically validated treatment. The inability to clearly show why EMDR works has resulted in its unfair categorization as a form of mesmerism.

HISTORY OF EYE-MOVEMENT DESENSITIZATION AND REPROCESSING

EMDR was founded serendipitously based on the personal experiences of its originator, Francine Shapiro, in the 1980s. Reportedly, while walking through a park contemplating disturbing personal issues, she noted an association between moving her eyes back and forth and a reduction in her emotional upset. She then is said to have paired these eye movements with other disturbing memories and noted a reduction in distress related to those memories. From these initial experiences she formally investigated the therapeutic value of eye movements and conducted a study of 22 traumatized individuals (Shapiro, 1989). Her results suggested that the pairing of eye movements with traumatic memories would reduce distress. Shapiro's technique not only involves reducing distress but also replacing negative beliefs, such as

http://dx.doi.org/10.1037/0000186-003
Alternative Therapies for PTSD: The Science of Mind–Body Treatments, by R. W. Motta

"I am a bad person" or "I am not worthy of love," with more positive self-views, such as "I did the best I could under the circumstances" or "I am a worthwhile individual."

Some suggested using in the EMDR label the term *desensitization*, which refers to a widely accepted behavioral psychology technique—known as *systematic desensitization*—of pairing progressively distressing and anxiety-provoking images with responses of relaxation. By pairing anxiety-producing imagery with relaxation, the imagery loses its power to evoke anxiety, and the client is thereby desensitized to the distressing imagery. In using a widely respected term and linking it to the new technique, the hope was that EMDR might become more acceptable to the academic and therapeutic communities, which tend to be slow in adjusting to and accepting new methods. Shapiro (2001), though, suggested that using the *desensitization* may have been a mistake (see, e.g., pp. xiv, 1). The term, as used in behavioral psychology, was not what was actually taking place in EMDR. As Shapiro (2001) stated, "If I had to do it over again, I might name it simply Reprocessing Therapy" (p. xiv).

Unfortunately, the inaccurate use of learning theory terminology like desensitization did not serve to arm EMDR against blisteringly critical attacks. Richard McNally (1999), a Harvard University–based psychotherapy researcher, drew similarities between EMDR and mesmerism and suggested that if EMDR has any effect, it is simply the result of client suggestibility. Thus, skepticism remains, and this is why EMDR is grouped under the "alternative therapy" rubric; in all fairness, though, those who value its having amassed a respectable level of empirical support would not consider EMDR as "alternative."

GENERAL FORMAT OF AN EYE-MOVEMENT DESENSITIZATION AND REPROCESSING SESSION

Although the specific techniques used in EMDR vary widely, in essence, the clinician asks the client to consider specific imagery associated with a personally experienced traumatic event and, in particular, the negative cognitions associated with the trauma, such as "I'm powerless," "I'm not worthwhile," and so forth. While engaging in this imagery, the client also visually tracks the therapist's index and middle finger—held together—as the therapist moves them laterally across the client's visual field. "The first set consists of 24 bidirectional movements, where a right-to-left-to-right shift equals one movement" (Shapiro, 2001, p. 67). Following the therapist's fingers across a swath of approximately 2 or 3 feet was the original procedure and perhaps currently is the most common. However, visually attending to alternating back-and-forth moving lights, attending to alternating auditory stimuli presented sequentially to each ear, and alternating tactile stimuli have subsequently been used.

Shapiro (2001) believed that the left–right alternation is a critical element in EMDR regardless of whether fingers, lights, or some other method is used.

When the set of movements is complete, the therapist then asks the client open-ended questions related to their experience, such as "What came up?" "What came to mind?" "How was that?" Unlike traditional psychotherapies, the clinician makes little attempt to guide, direct, or correct but simply asks the client to bring to mind a disturbing picture and the associated negative thoughts and any feelings or body sensations, and then to follow the therapist's fingers and report what thoughts, images, or emotions arise. Whatever it is that arises following the open-ended questioning, the therapist then reapplies the eye-tracking desensitization technique and allows that client to process this information. One continues this procedure until all disturbing material that was associated with the original trauma target has lost its disturbing quality. By pursuing an approach of asking the client what came to their mind because of the eye movements, the clinician is using the client's own associations and working through those rather than the clinician's own presumed associations.

Between sessions, the client practices previously taught self-management anxiety-reducing strategies, such as progressive muscle relaxation. The client eventually practices adaptive ways of construing events. So, for example, the rape victim might practice cognitions, such as "It was not my fault" or "I am a good person." These statements are subsequently subjected to the eye-movement procedure and, in that way, are presumably neurologically embedded and replace self-blame cognitions.

Emotions also become a target of the desensitization process. So, for example, the client may be asked to rate their negative affect, whether anxiety, anger, or depression, on a scale ranging from 1 (*minimal emotional concern*) to 10 (*extreme emotional distress*). If these emotions resist reduction through the original desensitization focus on cognitions, the emotions might then be subjected to the desensitization eye-movement procedure themselves.

The clinician also monitors body sensations. Traumatized people often have physical discomfort, such as neck pain, upset stomach, backaches, and headaches (van der Kolk, 2014). Observations of those who regularly provide EMDR treatment reveal that these sensations frequently are the last to be resolved. Consider the metaphor of a car moving down a dirt road. The passing of the car is a metaphorical passing of the distress over the traumatic experience. The dust that remains in the air represents the physical sensations, which linger even though the cognitive and emotional responses to the trauma have dramatically lessened. At this point, the clinician uses desensitization through eye movements to lessen the client's body distress. Again, the process is to have the client provide a rating of 1 to 10 of, for example, how much stomach upset they are experiencing. Use eye movements then helps reduce this distress.

As a final phase, the therapist asks the client to practice making positive self-statements and self-evaluations. For example, they may ask the client to focus on the positive images and thoughts of being a competent and worthwhile person who is able to deal with the "trials and tribulations" of life. The clinician obtains numerical ratings of the degree to which the client believes these positive statements and then engages the client in eye-movement exercises to help embed these newfound perceptions.

A Clinician's Memory Aid: TICES

A detailed description of the steps used in EMDR follows. When planning a course of treatment, it often is helpful for the practicing therapist to use the memory aid *TICES*: target memory, image, cognitions, emotions, and sensations. In addition, when planning an EMDR session, it is helpful for the therapist to know exactly what the trauma was or is; however, that information is not essential because EMDR sessions often start with images (I) or cognitions (C), or both, associated with the trauma and not the trauma itself. So, consider a rape situation (T). The image (I) might be that of an angry-looking man in a checkered shirt. The cognitions (C) might be "I can't do anything," "I am helpless," or "I am not worthwhile anymore." At this point, the therapist may start with either the *I* or *C* and begin making the bilateral finger movements across the client's visual field. After 20 to 30 cycles, the therapist may ask the client, "Okay, what came up?" Whatever arises is now the new stimulus for further eye movements (e.g., "Okay, now let's go with that thought: 'I am helpless'"), and a new round of bilateral movements begins. This process continues for about 90 minutes until the numerical ratings of believability, described later in this chapter, have moved in the desired direction, and the image or cognitions have lost their disruptive and disturbing quality.

The clinician deals with emotions (E), such as anger, fear, or sadness, in a similar manner as just described. They continue the bilateral movements until the disruptive emotions are resolved. Then the clinician subjects sensations (S), such as stomach tightness, back pain, neck stiffness, or any other physiological sensations associated with the traumatic experience, to the bilateral stimulation. This stimulation continues until the therapist observes a quieting of sensations. Some research (e.g., Rothbaum, 1997) reports that most single incident traumas are effectively managed in five or fewer session. Trauma of a developmental nature, such as emotional, physical, or sexual abuse, can take far longer because one's personality and outlook on life frequently are formed around, or significantly altered by, such traumas.

Automatic Self-Healing

EMDR advocates maintain that the nervous system and body, within which emotional and physical injuries take place, have a self-correcting, self-healing tendency (van der Kolk, 2014). The body attempts to heal a physical wound, such as a cut, and does so automatically. Sometimes the body requires assistance of antibiotics because of an infected wound; however, it is not the antibiotics that heal but the automatic body processes that are working to fight the infection. The same is said to be true of the mind. Traumatic experiences are isolated as images and sensations, and are kept from consciousness because of their disturbing nature. EMDR draws out these images and allows them to be processed by the thinking and aware parts of the brain: the cortex and especially the frontal lobes. From here, healing takes place automatically and progressively without apparent attention from the trauma sufferer.

This explanation of EMDR is, of course, conjecture. It is insightful conjecture but is nevertheless speculation. Other interventions, such as acupuncture (discussed in Chapter 7 of this volume), also highlight this self-healing tendency of body and mind. In acupuncture, the effect of needling is said to unblock healing energies of the body and mind, which then work automatically on an ongoing basis to resolve both physical and psychic pain. Both EMDR (Marich, 2011) and acupuncture (Brumbaugh, 1993) are said to have a low rate of relapse. Once the body and mind are healed, they usually do not "unheal." The initial sequestration of the trauma leads to an inability for healing processes to take place. The bilateral stimulation, whether eye movements or other forms of stimulation, reportedly bring cortical activation on line, and with it, automatic self-healing.

MECHANISMS OF ACTION

Clinicians naturally wish to know why a given treatment for a specific medical or psychological condition works. However, it may be less important that we understand how EMDR works than grasp its place as a viable alternative to other forms of psychotherapy that clients may not easily tolerate and therefore may avoid. EMDR is simply an alternative to traditional therapies and has amassed enough empirical support to be considered an empirically supported treatment by the Society of Clinical Psychology (Division 12) of the American Psychological Association (APA Presidential Task Force on Evidence-Based Practice, 2006), World Health Organization (2013), and International Society for Traumatic Stress Studies (Chemtob, Tolin, van der Kolk, & Pitman, 2000; Foa, Keane, & Friedman, 2000).

Other major organizations have not widely agreed on how EMDR works. Some have claimed that by making alternating eye movements and associating those movements with recollections of trauma, the traumatic memories are better integrated and "reprocessed" throughout the brain; this process is sometimes referred to as the *information-processing model* (Shapiro, 2001). The left–right movements presumably activate each of the cerebral hemispheres. This model of how EMDR works assumes that trauma memories are sequestered within the brain because of the posttraumatic stress disorder (PTSD) sufferer's inability to cope with them. This sequestration is the neurobiological equivalent of behavioral avoidance. The alternating eye movements are said to activate both sides of the brain, and because these movements are associated with trauma during EMDR, the trauma itself is neurologically processed bilaterally and no longer sequestered.

Another view is that the alternating eye movements are similar to what one sees in the rapid eye movement (REM) phase of sleep. Some have observed that problems are often resolved during sleep or at least seem less troublesome on awakening, and it is possible that this process of resolving problems is akin to what takes place in EMDR. For example, in an article detailing the neurological processes underlying utility of EMDR in treating PTSD, Stickgold (2002) stated

> that the repetitive redirecting of attention in EMDR induces a neurobiological state, similar to that of REM sleep, which is optimally configured to support the cortical integration of traumatic memories into general semantic networks. We suggest that this integration can then lead to a reduction in the strength of hippocampally mediated episodic memories of the traumatic event as well as well as the memories' associated, amygdala-dependent negative affect. (p. 61)

The translation of this complex statement is as follows: Episodic memories can be conceived of as discrete episodes related to trauma, such as specific events, sensations, images, or feelings that are stored in the hippocampus. These memories activate fear responses through the amygdala, and the memories are not integrated with one's overall conceptualization of the trauma and how one relates to it. The later integration, which follows from REM sleep or EMDR, would be considered to involve semantic memory as opposed to episodic memories, and these semantic memories are stored in the neocortex. Stickgold's interpretation may be considered the neurobiological equivalent of the information-processing model.

Are Eye Movements or Other Bilateral Stimulation Needed?

Another view is that eye movements, or other movements, per se are not central to the therapeutic process but rather serve as a distraction so that the traumatized client can keep images, sensations, and thoughts related to the trauma in awareness, without avoiding them, and thereby benefit from what turns out to be an exposure procedure (e.g., Barrowcliff, Gray, MacCulloch, Freeman, & MacCulloch, 2003; Rogers & Silver, 2002). This hypothesis might be called the distraction-exposure model of EMDR. Further research aimed at determining the validity of this hypothesis is needed.

Exposure as an explanatory mechanism is certainly one of the stances taken by those critical of the EMDR process. Because EMDR does not readily fit into known theoretical frameworks, it is forced in via the statement that it is simply a variant of known therapeutic procedures. Although one can reasonably argue that EMDR has an exposure component, something more seems to be involved. The surprisingly low rate of relapse said to be associated with EMDR (Marich, 2011) is not typically seen in exposure types of treatments. Relapse is common in exposure methods, especially when dealing with trauma. Some researchers have suggested that the low rate of relapse in EMDR is the result of the nervous system's having engaged in a self-healing process that does not then reverse itself (van der Kolk, 2014).

A number of provocative studies have compared the efficacy of standard EMDR with EMDR minus the eye movements (e.g., Davidson & Parker, 2001). These studies essentially found no difference between EMDR with and without eye movements. It could be argued that removing the eye movements makes EMDR a form of prolonged exposure (PE) therapy in that clients are asked to repeatedly recount elements of their trauma. Most who are able to endure PE do get better. The problem is that when one moves from laboratory studies to real-world application, most trauma sufferers will not stay with PE because it is too aversive (Morris, 2015). An interesting aside is that almost 85% of therapists also do not do any form of exposure therapy (Zayfert et al., 2005). So, between client avoidance of treatments involving anxiety-provoking confrontation of their fears and traumas, and lack of usage by therapists, exposure-based therapies have serious limitations as far as treatments for PTSD are concerned. Again, it is the aversion to PTSD treatments involving exposure to traumatic material that has opened the door to alternative therapies that clients presumably can tolerate more easily.

I am not arguing that there is or is not an exposure aspect to EMDR but to maintain that EMDR is nothing more than exposure does not seem to square with observations of treatment outcomes. Although no one knows for certain how EMDR works, empirical studies have shown that it is effective in dealing with PTSD. Carlson, Chemtob, Rusnak, Hedlund, and Muraoka (1998) claimed a 78% effectiveness rate in treating combat-related PTSD. Maybe it is not as important to know why an intervention works than knowing it does. In a historical note, van der Kolk (2014) wryly pointed out that in regard to the history of penicillin, "almost four decades passed between the discovery of its antibiotic properties by Alexander Fleming in 1928 and the final elucidation of its mechanisms in 1995" (p. 262). Aspirin was also widely used for many years, even though it was unclear why it worked. EMDR seems to work for reasons that are not entirely clear, just as aspirin once did.

Despite the demonstrated utility of EMDR in treating PTSD, the majority of veterans of recent wars in Iraq and Afghanistan do not seek it or any other kind of treatment for PTSD (Hoge et al., 2004). Veterans are notoriously treatment avoidant. Some of this avoidance can be laid at the door of perception, that is, help-seeking may not fit within the training and self-image context of what it means to be a military combatant. It is also highly likely that many forms of therapy for PTSD, no matter how well intended, provoke such extreme levels of anxiety that veterans avoid them at all costs.

Has EMDR shown itself to be more effective than PE? No, according to Rothbaum, Astin, and Marsteller (2005). EMDR, though, seems to work more quickly and is less likely to show relapse. However, it might be argued that exposure protocols used in research often devote sessions to completing assessment measures and provide participants with a rationale for uncomfortable exposure, and it is these factors that make PE seem to take longer. If you, the reader, are getting the sense that for every argument supporting or not supporting a particular form of therapy there are counter arguments, then you can see why addressing therapeutic effectiveness is such a thorny issue.

If Eye-Movement Desensitization and Reprocessing Is No More Effective Than Exposure Therapies, Why Bother With It?

This interesting question goes to the heart of why alternative therapies for PTSD exist at all. It is certainly important for clinicians to know whether a given form of therapy works, but, again, if a therapy is difficult for a client to tolerate, they will simply avoid it, and it therefore will be of no use. PE, a mainstay in the treatment of PTSD, requires repetitively revisiting traumatic experiences, and by confronting them, they lose some of their power to disrupt one's life. It may very well be that the reason that EMDR has found a place in the treatment of trauma is that it is comparatively easier to tolerate than PE. Unlike conventional exposure treatment, EMDR spends little time revisiting the original trauma. The trauma itself—or the images associated with the trauma—is certainly the starting point, but the focus of EMDR is on stimulating and opening up the associative process (van der Kolk, 2014). In a typical EMDR session, the therapist encourages the client to pursue thoughts, images, sensations, or emotions that arise following a series of passes of the therapist's fingers before the client's eyes. The client is not cajoled, implored, or encouraged to maintain a focus on the distressing traumatic event per se, as is the case in PE.

However, that EMDR does deal with traumatic material, no matter how indirectly, does give some clients pause. Dealing with trauma is anxiety provoking. In many instances, dealing with trauma directly or indirectly activates emotional avoidance and a desire to distance oneself from the therapy and the therapist.

Eight Phases of Eye-Movement Desensitization and Reprocessing Treatment

EMDR is a somewhat involved form of intervention that Shapiro (2001) broke down into eight detailed phases. Some authors have argued that not all of these steps are actually necessary, nor is the rigid adherence to Shapiro's assessment and evaluation procedures needed for successful treatment (e.g., Marich, 2011). It may be that Shapiro (2001) developed a rigid set of procedures and assessment protocols to mitigate the vitriolic resistance that this ostensibly unorthodox procedure seemed to evoke from professionals and academics. Nevertheless, the stages of treatment are described in the sections that follow.

Phase 1: Client History and Treatment Planning

People who have been traumatized usually have a specific painful memory or memories of the traumatic event. During a combat experience, one may have an embedded and persistent panicky feeling associated with a combat engagement. This discomforting emotion arises with memories of combat.

A rape victim may recall the overwhelming anxiety and violence of the attack. These images or episodes are the focal point or *targets*—to use Stickgold's (2002) term—that form the beginnings of the EMDR session. Strangely, it may not actually be necessary for the clinician to obtain a specific and detailed description of the traumatic event or events. This deemphasizing of trauma specifics can be helpful in allaying the intensity of anxiety associated with the trauma. During EMDR, the trauma victim focuses on a target, which could be a feeling such as helplessness, feeling diminished, believing that one is worthless, the foul breath of the rapist, or some other episode associated with the trauma.

During the initial stage of the EMDR procedure, one focuses on the target, and when the first phase of eye movements is complete, the therapist asks, "What came to mind?" It is the processing of the target and everything associated with it that forms the mainstay of treatment. During this phase of treatment, the clinician attempts to obtain all relevant information, including family, educational, and employment history; preexisting modes of coping with stress; and emotional resources. At all points in treatment, the clinician is supportive, encouraging, and understanding, and makes every effort to not push the client to the point of evoking a response of avoidance or aversion.

Phase 2: Preparation

In the preparation phase, the clinician works on establishing rapport and explaining the details of treatment to the client so that the client is fully informed and not in any way surprised by the treatment process. Another important phase of preparation is teaching relaxation so that one feels they have a means of addressing any apprehensions that may arise as a result of treatment. The clinician can use anxiety-reducing methods, such as progressive muscle relaxation, practicing the use of calling up serene and pleasant images, training in yoga, or meditation. In essence, the client learns coping skills to help them manage the anxiety that is likely to arise as they confront traumatic episodes.

Phase 3: Assessment

The purpose of the assessment phase is to establish a baseline response to the trauma memory and image or images associated with that memory. It is this response to the image or target that is the initial focus of EMDR. The therapist asks the client to indicate the specific maladaptive beliefs associated with this target image. For example, the rape victim may hold beliefs, such as "I am worthless," "I am at fault for not having fought back," or "I am bad, and no one would want me." The client then generates alternative positive cognitions, such as "I am a worthwhile and valuable person" or "I did the best I could under extremely frightening conditions." The clinician then assesses the validity of this positive cognition (i.e., validity of cognition [VoC]) on a scale of 1 (*being not valid or unbelievable*) to 7 (*being believable*). One of the goals of EMDR is to bring this rating from a low of 1 or 2 to a high of 6 or 7.

Next, the therapist assesses the emotional intensity of the trauma image or images using the Subjective Units of Distress Scale (Wolpe & Lazarus, 1966), which ranges from 1 (*none or almost none*) to 10 (*maximum or most intense*). As with the VoC measure, the goal is to significantly reduce the level of experienced distress, in this case, to a 1 or 2. The therapist asks the client to identify where in the body they feel the distressing sensations to give a numerical rating to, for example, the stomach or neck distress. The assessment phase provides a quantitative way of assessing progress in EMDR therapy.

Phase 4: Desensitization and Reprocessing

During this phase, the client keeps the target of trauma in mind along with associated sensations, images, and cognitions while the clinician moves their fingers, held approximately a foot in front of the client's eyes, back and forth approximately 20 to 30 times, and the client follows the fingers with their eyes. Alternative approaches include using light bars to present alternating lights that the client visually tracks and that require left-and-right-eye movements, auditory stimuli that alternate from ear to ear, alternate hand taps, and pressure cuffs that alternate pulses from one wrist to the next. While the client follows the back-and-forth movements, the therapist asks them to clear their mind and let go of the trauma target, take a deep breath, and report anything that may have come up, whether images, memories, sensations, or something else. Usually, a minimum direction from the therapist is called for, but whatever the client says has come up because of the first round of eye movements serves as the target for the next set of eye movements for similar sets of stimulation. This process of having one idea, image, or feeling serve as the stimulus for the next is referred to as *adaptive information processing* in the EMDR parlance. The therapist encourages the client to move forward in this manner to desensitize each item that comes up with the use of the eye movement process.

Phase 5: Installation of Positive Cognition

The fifth phase emphasizes the replacement of negative, maladaptive cognitions with positive, adaptive ones. This process takes place after the negative affect, as measured using the Subjective Units of Distress Scale (Wolpe & Lazarus, 1966), has been reduced to near zero. So, for example, once the emotional distress has been reduced through desensitization and reprocessing, the person who was sexually abused might use a cognition like "I have the capability to prevent this from happening" to replace "I am powerless." The positive cognition is associated with the memory of the abuse and subjected to the eye-movement desensitization procedure. The clinician then continues with the desensitization and reprocessing using the eye-movement procedure until the VoC reaches a level of 7 (i.e., *believable*). Although the positive cognition might be one that the client identified during the assessment phase, it could also be one that emerged spontaneously during the reprocessing procedure. The clinician should continue to engage in the reprocessing while the client practices associating the positive cognition with the previously identified traumatic images. In doing so, a general reduction in negative affect and negative perceptions continues to evolve.

Some clients may be unable to attain a VoC of 7 and claim, "I don't deserve to be completely free of self-blame" or "I can't give a 7 until my significant other validates that I have overcome my negativism." If these or similar views occur, the therapist then treats them as targets of desensitization and reprocessing, and identifies new positive cognitions, such as "I do deserve to be free of self-blame as I've done nothing wrong" or "I don't need the opinion of others to validate my worth." What the clinician is seeking is to have positive cognitions become associated with other thoughts that might surround the traumatic experience. Traditional learning theorists might use the term *generalization* to describe this associative process of the linking of positive cognitions to other trauma-relevant cognitions. EMDR theorists prefer the term *association*.

Regardless of terminology, trauma is typically associated with cognitions of powerlessness, inability, and worthlessness. The critical installation of positive cognitions that emphasize having the ability to choose to alter the negative events in which the client found themselves and the accompanying improvement in self-view are crucial to successful treatment using EMDR—or any other form of treatment, for that matter. People who are traumatized are disempowered and feel victimized. The installation of positive cognitions and their association with the trauma are oriented toward reversing these negative consequences of trauma and empowering the client.

Phase 6: Body Scan

After the installation of positive cognitions, the therapist asks the client to simultaneously hold in mind the trauma target and the positive cognition, and to scan the body mentally from head to toe. If the client detects tension in any part of the body—such detection is not at all unusual—these body sensations are subjected to successive sets of eye- (or other) movement desensitization. Presumably, the body mirrors psychological trauma, and although these body sensations often resolve automatically with EMDR treatment, sometimes they persist and have to be dealt with by addressing them with successive sets of desensitization.

Phase 7: Closure

This phase involves debriefing the client at the end of an EMDR session and preparing them for any negative (or positive) images, feelings, or cognitions that might arise between sessions. The clinician emphasizes self-management of stress in the form of access to relaxation audiotapes or videos. The client can maintain journals or logs to document anything that may come up. They must be assured that because difficult material has been covered during the session, difficult memories might arise between sessions. By documenting in writing the things that have surfaced, the client is empowered in managing their distress. Similarly, by having access to relaxation audio and videotapes, the client is similarly empowered.

Phase 8: Reevaluation

At the beginning of each session, the clinician attempts to assess where the client stands with regard to the VoC, Subjective Units of Distress Scale (Wolpe & Lazarus, 1966), and body scan relevant to the material that the client has processed. In addition, the clinician attempts to determine the degree to which that processed material has generalized to the "real world" of the client. Does the client see changes in their views and their behavior as a result of treatment? It is possible that changes in the client's behavior have evoked changes in the reactions of those close to him or her. If so and conflicts have arisen, the clinician must deal with these issues for the client's benefit. One might consider the reevaluation phase an objective information-gathering step that helps the clinician and the client move ahead in a productive manner.

CASE EXAMPLE: STARTING EYE-MOVEMENT DESENSITIZATION AND REPROCESSING WITH A TROUBLED PROFESSIONAL

Ronald is a chemist who works for the U.S. Drug Enforcement Administration in New York City. He spends much of his workdays testing and identifying samples of illicit drugs. Despite his obvious intelligence and capability, Ronald is incredibly self-doubting and courteous to the point of being obsequious. His uncertainty and need for assurance can be traced back to a troubled childhood in which his mother was alternatively remote, critical, and castigating and, at other times, doting and overly close. Ronald describes her as bipolar. His biological father was a dentist who left the home when Ronald was 3 years old. His mother remarried a man whom Ronald described as explosive, punitive, alcoholic, and remote. When he was asked which of his childhood experiences troubled him the most, he mentioned a trip to Florida with his mother during which she criticized him and made it clear for the entire trip what a disappointment he was. He was 9 years old and felt trapped with his mother and her barrage of critiques. This feeling of entrapment is a common element in trauma cases.

After explaining the basics to Ronald, our EMDR session started with an image of sitting in the back seat on the Florida trip feeling confined, diminished, and miserable. A particular focus was on his self-views of being incompetent.

After the first set of alternating eye movements, what came up was his mother's variability of moods from loving to emotionally abusive. Next were memories of his stepfather whom he detested and avoided. Then images emerged of how school had provided a haven of safety where he was not abused and critiqued. Through a period of three sessions, Ronald came to the position that although he was the recipient of criticism by both his mother and stepfather, it was likely that they were troubled souls who vented their difficulties onto him. He came to see that their behavior toward him spoke more of their own deficits than of his. This was an important realization for Ronald, after which he seemed visibly less distressed and far more insightful as to the nature of his difficulties.

Ronald will continue to need help for a myriad of problems, including relationship difficulties, all of which are rooted in a troubled childhood. Nevertheless, EMDR did play a valuable role in facilitating the development of insight into the nature of his difficulties. In this case, EMDR served as a tool that helped overcome a roadblock. It did not serve to resolve all of this client's difficulties, but Ronald saw it as highly effective in that it helped him put some tormenting memories behind him so he could move on in therapy.

CONTROVERSIES

Undoubtedly, EMDR is controversial, perhaps because of the peculiar eye-movement element of the treatment and the difficulty meshing these movements with traditional learning theory that underlies cognitive behavior therapy (CBT). It is also controversial in that it claims to treat PTSD far more quickly than CBT methods, and some clinicians claim one session "cures." Practicing therapists are well aware that one-session cures are few and far between, but EMDR does deal with a specific trauma, such as a car accident, fairly quickly (i.e., in a few sessions). Traumas that are developmental in nature, such as those precipitated by childhood physical and sexual abuse or emotional neglect, may require years of treatment.

Another controversy has to do with the mechanism or mechanisms of action of EMDR. At times, therapists simply don't know why an intervention works. For example, as we learned in the case of aspirin mentioned earlier, we simply did not know for many years why it was effective in treating various physical illnesses. If we are honest with ourselves, we might have to admit that not knowing why an intervention works is likely to be the case far more often than knowing. There seems to be a self-correcting or self-healing component to EMDR. Once the right conditions are in place, the nervous system seems to move in the direction of repair much like the physical system does. EMDR appears to activate some form of a self-correcting, neurobiological rebalancing process.

Many of the alternative interventions I address in other chapters have this characteristic of activating a self-healing process. Data exist showing that the various alternative interventions work in alleviating trauma symptoms, but it is unclear why this finding is so. Physical exercise is a good example. It has clear benefits in lessening the distress of anxiety, depression, and other emotional concerns, but researchers have not identified a specific mechanism or reason why these benefits occur. Much of modern medicine conforms to this model. Physicians may be able to provide the environment for the body to heal, but it is the body itself that brings the healing about.

Despite these controversies, EMDR is a valuable tool in that it addresses trauma in a way that is less trying to both client and therapist than procedures such as PE. In PE, the client and the therapist repeatedly go over highly distressing scenes, such as rape, images of war, or terrible atrocities. This process is difficult for anyone. However, in all fairness, EMDR, although not as aversive and difficult to tolerate as PE, may evoke strong emotions related to traumatic experiences, too. As a result, many might also consider it somewhat difficult to tolerate. Comprehensive data are not available regarding the tolerability of EMDR.

LIMITATIONS

A client of mine recently encountered the outcome of his beloved son's having shot himself in the head with a shotgun after having taken lysergic acid diethylamide, or LSD. Hearing the blast, the young man's father came into the bedroom to find his son on the floor, his brain sitting next to his head. Engaging in PE or even EMDR for such an experience seems both unthinkable and inhumane, especially at this early phase of treatment. The outcome in cases such as this is that both clients and clinicians tend to avoid exposure treatments. If a treatment is available that lessens the pain or time required for the client get better, that is the treatment of choice. To quote Rothbaum (1997), "The quickest, least painful effective treatment is the most desirable" (p. 319). The hope is that alternative treatments for PTSD, such as EMDR and others I cover in later chapters, will turn out to be both quicker and less painful than traditional approaches for many forms of psychological trauma.

Another limitation of EMDR treatment is that it is somewhat complex. Clinicians would be well advised to seek specialized training in its multistage process. It is unlikely that one can simply pick up a book and, from a description of the EMDR procedure, be able to begin treating clients or to engage in self-treatment. The untrained practitioner has the potential to either excessively elevate the client's anxiety or simply be ineffective. In either case, the client might be so discouraged that they no longer seek treatment for their trauma.

The use of procedures oriented toward asking clients to revisit aspects of their trauma is hard on therapists who have traditionally been trained to alleviate suffering and distress, let alone difficult for their clients. PE therapy and, to a lesser extent, EMDR emphasize repeatedly confronting the actual trauma experience (PE) or cognitions, sensations, and emotions associated with the trauma (EMDR). However, the hope of affecting a "cure" for PTSD with low rates of relapse is what draws increasing numbers of clinicians to this mode of treatment.

That EMDR does not fit easily into known theoretical frameworks and that there seems to be no widely agreed on explanation of how it works has hampered its acceptance. I know of no tabulation of the number of psychologists who are trained in and use EMDR, but I personally know of only one or two out of hundreds. It is simply not a mainstream form of treatment.

STRENGTHS

EMDR has shown itself to be an effective treatment for PTSD in many cases, and its official label as an empirically supported treatment given by major professional organizations bodes well for its future success. It is included in this volume as an effective "alternative" only because it is not a mainstream form of treatment. The seemingly low rate of relapse reported by the majority of EMDR practitioners is somewhat unusual in the world of psychotherapy. It does give one the impression that EMDR may set the stage for a neuro-psychological self-healing process. Although this explanation may seem fanciful to some, it is a widely accepted process in the world of physical injury. Why couldn't the same occur with psychological injury? It is an interesting aside that acupuncture also claims to stimulate self-healing, self-correcting, and rebalancing processes, as I detail in Chapter 7. EMDR has provided relief to numerous veterans and to those who have experienced and survived rape, accident, terrorist attack, and natural disaster. That is justification enough for its use whether it is mainstream or not.

SUMMARY

Clinicians have used EMDR for more than 30 years in treating trauma. When it first arrived on the therapeutic scene, it was greeted with a high level of suspicion and skepticism. Some viewed it—and many continue to do so—as little more than a fad in which the impact likely resulted from placebo effects. Now it is seen as having a high level of empirical support, and the American Psychological Association accepted EMDR as an empirically supported treatment for PTSD. Although the technique continues to have its skeptics, the empirical support for EMDR is compelling.

3

Yoga for PTSD

An increasing trend is for those who have experienced trauma and post-traumatic stress disorder (PTSD), such as war veterans, rape victims, and natural disaster survivors, to turn to yoga for relief of their distress (Jackson, 2014). The reason is perhaps simple: Yoga does not demand that one confront thoughts, images, or memories of the trauma. Thus, the anxiety and threat often fostered by traditional psychotherapies are reduced with a consequent reduction in avoidance of treatment. No single definition of yoga exists, but in Sanskrit the term means "union" or "connection" and can be said to imply a connection to greater awareness in living or a union or yoking of body and mind (Kaley-Isley, Peterson, Fischer, & Peterson, 2010). Yoga has been practiced in various forms for more than 5,000 years, approximately 20 different types are practiced in the United States, and yoga has in all about 80,000 stances or postures (*asanas*; Emerson & Hopper, 2011). The Vedas and Upanishads are considered to be some of the earliest texts encompassing yoga practice and sacred literature in Hinduism. Yoga grew out of a region now known as India and Pakistan. Today, one can find yoga classes in nearly any American city, and approximately 16 million people practice regularly (Emerson & Hopper, 2011).

Most forms of yoga involve a combination of breathing practice (*pranayama*), stretches (*asanas*), relaxation (*savasana*), and meditation, although meditation is frequently used in and of itself as a treatment for psychological trauma. *Meditation* requires intentionally clearing the mind of its wandering thoughts and developing an evolving focus on the present moment. In the case of yoga, this focus on the present often involves a focus on the postures, the effort

http://dx.doi.org/10.1037/0000186-004
Alternative Therapies for PTSD: The Science of Mind–Body Treatments, by R. W. Motta

required to hold them, and the balance needed to do them well. Ongoing and constant practice is required for one to get hold of mind wandering and to develop a focus on the present moment, but this process is aided by a focus on posture and balance in yoga. Such practice is particularly true for the trauma survivor who spends a great deal of time reliving the traumatic past. One might consider PTSD as a disorder that specifically entails living in or dwelling in the past. These individuals are often two people: one presents the public image; we see this person at work, school, or social events. The other is the unseen frightened and brutalized person; this person is the weary, distrustful, on-guard, hypervigilant survivor who is hidden from view but very much present. These two selves live side by side. For the traumatized individual, the brutal and torturous past is always present. One of the goals of yoga is to be fully present as one person, one awareness, and in the here and now, and not a shadow reflection of the past.

A question that might be reasonably asked is, Why should the specific techniques that are used in yoga work at all in helping people and particularly traumatized people? There is not a generally agreed on answer to this question because yoga has many components, but one possibility is that what we refer to as "mind" and to "body" are actually inextricably linked, and this unity is supported by a great deal of research (e.g., Pert, 1999). If the body can be moved to let go of its distress and tension as in yoga practice, there's a good chance this release will impact mental and emotional states in a positive and calming way. An anxious mind seems unable to exist in a relaxed body (Jacobson, 1938). The Latin expression *mens sana in copore sano* is apropos here and is roughly translated to "a healthy mind in a healthy body" ("*Mens Sana in Corpore Sano*," n.d.). The expression is often used in educational and exercise contexts to highlight that physical well-being goes hand in hand with emotional and psychological well-being. Physical tranquility is yoked to mental/emotional peace and vice versa, thus, different methods of yoga might emphasize either physical ease or mental tranquility in its ongoing practice.

I do not attempt here to advocate for one form of yoga because many forms exist and can involve variations in the speed and depth of breathing and use of the mouth, nostrils, and throat, as well as different forms of stretching, postures, room temperature, meditations, and so on, reportedly producing differing psychological and physical results. Some forms of yoga place a greater emphasis on postures and balance; some, on meditative procedures; and some emphasize all of these. Possible critical elements or essential mechanisms of yoga include self-regulation (e.g., Dick, Niles, Street, DiMartino, & Mitchell, 2014), interoceptive awareness (e.g., van der Kolk, 2006), and stress physiology (e.g., Riley & Park, 2015). But, clearly, researchers do not agree:

> On a biochemical and physiological level, previous research has shown that yoga relaxes chronic muscle tension, restores natural diaphragmatic breathing, improves oxygen absorption and carbon dioxide elimination, increases alpha and theta brain waves, and regulates the thalamus at an optimum level. (Weintraub, 2012, p. 14)

Although views of what yoga does for an individual may differ, let us take the position that yoga involves an integration of bodily and mental/emotional states, and an awareness of this integration. Trauma typically eventuates in a separation from one's mental/emotional states because traumatic experiences are too painful to endure. Yoga attempts to unite or yoke body and mind, and in that way, it combats the negative, separating effects of trauma.

YOGA AND TRAUMA

In the description of PTSD in Chapter 1, I stated that the disorder meets a series of criteria as set forth in the current edition of the *Diagnostic and Statistical Manual of Mental Disorders* (fifth ed.; American Psychiatric Association, 2013). I also indicated that PTSD frequently entails an alienation from one's sense of self and a wary and suspicious view of one's environment. Often PTSD sufferers hunker down emotionally and withdraw into themselves. This seems a natural self-protective reaction to having been severely frightened, or in fear for one's life, or both. This hunkering down is so basic, so survival oriented, that issues like self-knowledge, self-awareness, and introspection are replaced by a far more important and basic mandate: survival. This primacy of the survival instinct frequently results in people's not being in touch with themselves and who they are. Many suffer from a condition known as *alexithymia* that is characterized by an inability to identify and describe one's emotions. This inability results in difficulty understanding the emotions of others and a consequent social insensitivity and awkwardness. Alexithymia is often seen in Holocaust survivors (Krystal & Krystal, 1988) and in traumatized veterans. PTSD results in a cutting off of one's thoughts and feelings because they are so painful. However, the body keeps the score (van der Kolk, 2014) and continues to register the pain. The practice of yoga is aimed at reintegration. It is a reconnecting of one's thoughts and feelings with one's body. It entails becoming increasingly familiar with one's thoughts, feelings, and behaviors, and consequently being better attuned to others.

This reacquaintance with one's feelings is no easy matter for the traumatized individual; as a result, specific approaches generally alluded to as trauma-sensitive yoga have come about (e.g., Emerson & Hopper, 2011). The inner turmoil of traumatized individuals may present as tension in the shoulders, a crushing sensation in the chest, or a burning in the abdomen. The body has registered the extremes of emotional distress with bodily felt pains and agonies. The traumatized person makes every effort to avoid and create distance from both the emotional and physical pain, and it is this avoidance (i.e., not dealing with the issues) that maintains the distress. The integrative properties of yoga can certainly help to unite body and mind, but the survival-motivated avoidance tendencies in those with PTSD work against accepting this integration. The great benefits of yoga as an alternative to traditional forms of therapy are that it is holistic in its mind–body inclusion and that one does not need to directly confront their trauma to reap the benefits of yoga.

Trauma-Sensitive Yoga Versus Standard Yoga Practice

Before explaining the differences between these two forms of yoga, it is necessary to understand that most forms of traumatic experience and PTSD involve some type of reduction in one's choices and of being forced to endure extremely difficult circumstances. The rape victim is attacked, held, and sexually and physically brutalized. The military combatant encounters situations involving an imminent threat to one's life and without much chance of escape. The combatant follows orders and is allowed few options in choosing the dangers they must confront. In the Introduction, I offered an example of orders that conflicted with my division's attempts to stay alive during the Vietnam War. The physically and sexually abused child is powerless and fearful of fighting back. The captured military person is confined and tormented physically and mentally. Trauma and PTSD most often involve some form of confinement, powerlessness, and extremes of fear.

Now consider that most *standard forms of yoga* are directed, guided, and scripted. One is not free to choose one's postures. The yoga teacher selects them. Often, a yoga instructor will move about the room and physically guide the participant by touching them and moving them into the "correct" position. This perceived reduction in choice and of being touched while being instructed and guided sets off alarm bells for the person with PTSD. A response of extreme aversion and avoidance reflexively comes to the surface. Survival mode is activated, and the yoga trainee either flees or chooses to never return for additional sessions. Thus, alternative approaches to teaching yoga are needed, especially for those suffering from PTSD.

Trauma-sensitive yoga involves a decreased emphasis on getting the positions just right. It involves virtually no touching and a deemphasis on guidance. The yoga instructor makes it clear that there is no "right" way to engage in the postures. If directions are called for, the instructor presents them as suggestions only and makes it clear that the participant does not need to engage in the postures as prescribed. Even the verbiage of the session is altered. Rather than saying, "Sit in this way," one might consider saying, "Allow yourself to sit this way if it is comfortable for you." The emphasis is on choice, and this choice might even extend so far as scheduling the session (e.g., "Do you think a 9, 10, or 11 o'clock class would work for you?" or "Which would you prefer?"). Again, here, the emphasis is on placing control in the hands of the trauma victim and less so with the teacher. It is helpful to inform the yoga participant that they can leave the session at any time, that there will be no touching, and that the instructor is available to discuss any aspect of the training that the participant would like. It is important for the instructor to emphasize that people vary in their flexibility and capability of assuming postures, so participants have no chance of doing it "wrong." If the participant wants direction, they are free to ask for it. If the instructor feels strongly that a posture be done in a particular way, it is incumbent on the instructor to present this posture in as nondirective a manner as they can.

It is possible that the aversion to any form of yoga that is perceived as directive and confining serves to activate the fleeing response and that this aversion cannot be overcome regardless how nondirective the instruction. In such cases, I suggest that the trauma victim consider the use of CDs, DVDs, or videos that one can find on YouTube. In these situations, the trauma victim can choose the type of material they might want to experience. They can go at their own pace and will not receive any form of correction. Nevertheless, it is important for the clinician to be mindful of the all-encompassing influence of the traumatic experience. The postures and breathing exercises, although liberating and freeing, have the potential to put the trauma sufferer in touch with their painful emotions and memories, which can bring on a panicky flight response. From this, you, the reader, can gain an appreciation of the power and influence that PTSD has over the trauma victim and the critical need to move slowly and judiciously when treating trauma.

Specific Trauma-Sensitive Yoga Programs

Yoga uses a variety of techniques and methods designed to increase awareness and a sense of control and integration. A popular yoga-meditative practice often used with PTSD sufferers is called *iRest*, or *integrative restoration*, "which is a modern-day variation of the ancient practice of yoga nidra" (Miller, 2015, p. 2). The approach places a greater emphasis on meditative approaches and deep relaxation, and less emphasis on postures, and it appears to have achieved wide acceptance for treating military and nonmilitary-based PTSD. The program iRest yoga *nidra*—in Sanskrit, *nidra* refers to changing states of consciousness— "teaches self-care skills for healing and resolving symptoms of PTSD" (Miller, 2015, pp. 18–19). iRest comprises 10 tools (Miller, 2015):

- affirming one's mission,
- noting one's intentions,
- examining one's inner resources,
- engaging in body awareness and relaxation,
- being aware of one's breath,
- recognizing and accepting negative and positive thoughts,
- welcoming opposites of thought (i.e., learning how to respond to both negative and positive thoughts),
- appreciating inner joy,
- appreciating one's existence, and
- appreciating one's self in relation to others (i.e., one's wholeness).

As a result of research sponsored by the U.S. Department of Defense (Miller, 2015), iRest programs are being brought to U.S. Department of Veterans Affairs facilities, active duty military facilities, and medical facilities around North America.

According to Miller (2007), the purpose of engaging in regular iRest yoga practice is "to induce deep relaxation throughout the body and mind, eliminate stress, overcome insomnia, solve personal and interpersonal problems, resolve trauma, and to neutralize and overcome anxiety, fear, anger and depression" (p. 1). Once tensions and muscular strain abate, further practice "[provides] us with guidelines for investigating and going beyond self-limiting beliefs and conditions in order to break free of restrictive patterns so that we can live a contented life, free of conflict, anxiety, fear dissatisfaction and suffering" (p. 171).

Another popular form of yoga used with military veterans with PTSD and traumatic brain injury, as well as other traumatized groups is Yoga for Warriors (Bender, 2014). Yoga for Warriors relies heavily on *ashtanga yoga*, which emphasizes physically demanding and strenuous poses that move rapidly from one to another and are believed to fit in with the modes of training and experience of military combatants. Unlike iRest, which emphasizes meditation, Yoga for Warriors places much heavier emphasis on stances and postures, breathing practices, and movement. Yoga Warriors International, which seems to have spun off from the original Yoga for Warriors, places emphasis of this form of yoga primarily on the development of a sense of control and a secure connection with the present moment by relying heavily on postures. This emphasis on posture and control is in direct contrast with what is experienced by traumatized individuals who feel out of control and lack a secure connection to anything. Military personnel are trained to be highly focused externally and to be vigilant of what the "enemy" might be doing. Yoga for Warriors takes that trained skill of vigilance and strength and turns it inward so that the trauma sufferer becomes more aware of and attuned to their emotions, thoughts, and behaviors. Although the emphasis on posture and balance of Yoga for Warriors contrasts with the primarily meditative and relaxation approaches used in the iRest training program, they may share a focus on the present, including one's own functioning. Whereas trauma eventuates in feelings of being out of control, yoga in its various forms emphasizes control, focus, and being present whether the practices are primarily meditative or postural. Yoga emphasizes an integration of body and mind, and, as such, is "its own form of meditation, which, of course, all yoga is when understood properly" (Kabat-Zinn, 1990, p. 108). If popularity of an intervention is a measure of either utility or effectiveness in treating PTSD, yoga is a valuable resource for those suffering from this disorder.

Types of Yoga

Approximately 20 types of yoga exist in the United States alone, and this may be a conservative estimate. Finding the "right" form of yoga is somewhat similar to finding the "right" form of exercise. It is all up to individual taste, but it would seem that the "right" form is the one that an individual is likely to do on an ongoing basis. So, matching individual needs with type of yoga is equally, if not more, important than finding the "right" yoga. Some traumatized people prefer yoga approaches that are less directive and have fewer demands that poses and positions be executed precisely. Others might prefer strenuous approaches that leave a sense of having completed a serious workout, and in that way, they may experience a sense of emotional release. Some of the more popular forms of yoga include the following (Emerson & Hopper, 2011):

- *Hatha yoga*, which emphasizes body postures and balance, and is said to be for beginners;

- *Vinyasa yoga*, a form that links movement and breath in a dancelike, fast-moving pace;

- *Iyengar yoga*, which places emphasis on precise body alignment;

- *Ashtanga yoga*, a form that uses six series of specifically sequenced yoga poses;

- *Bikram yoga*, which uses two breathing exercises and 26 poses in a room of 105 °F and 40% humidity for 90 minutes;

- *Kundalini yoga*, a form emphasizing repetitive physical exercises coupled with intense breath work;

- *Hot yoga*, which is similar to Bikram yoga but not confined to 26 poses;

- *Yin yoga*, a form intended to calm and balance mind and body, and that is the opposite of ashtanga in that participants hold Yin poses for several minutes at a time; and

- *Restorative yoga*, which emphasizes meditation and a mellow, slow-moving practice with longer poses and also emphasizes meditation. This is the type of yoga noted earlier that some would advocate as useful in dealing with PTSD.

Significant overlap exists between yoga and meditation, which I cover in Chapter 4, and some would take the position that yoga is a form of movement meditation (e.g., Boccio, 2004).

YOGA RESOURCES FOR CLINICIANS AND TRAUMA SUFFERERS

A number of texts that specifically address the use of yoga for treating trauma can be of value to those who suffer from and those who treat trauma. The first is *Overcoming Trauma Through Yoga: Reclaiming Your Body* (Emerson & Hopper, 2011). Although the book focuses on specific yoga practices that one can use in the treatment of trauma, it emphasizes four themes that each yoga session should touch on when dealing with trauma: (a) experiencing the present moment, (b) making choices, (c) taking effective action, and (d) creating rhythms.

Recall that PTSD may be viewed as a disorder of not being present. The attention needed to engage in and maintain prescribed yoga postures necessitates experiencing the present moment, that is, focusing on the present and having an awareness of sensations of the body in the present moment. Attention to breathing also directs one's attention to the present.

Another theme is making choices. Trauma involves the inability to act effectively to escape the traumatic situation. In trauma-sensitive yoga, the instructor encourages the participant to enact choices, such as how far they wish to take a given posture, how little or how much discomfort they are willing to endure, whether to engage in a particular posture at all, or whether they wish to modify a given posture to their liking. The practice of making choices runs counter to the experience of entrapment and lack of choice that are essential elements of trauma.

A related element is taking effective action. Given that trauma victims do not seem to be able to escape the rape or the combat situation, for example, trauma sensitive yoga encourages participants to inform the instructor on changes they would want to see in the session, whether it be room temperature, the pace of the session, or the opening or closing of windows.

Another element involves creating rhythms. At the Child and Family Trauma Institute that I direct and in my clinical practice, trauma survivors report being out of synch with others, of living in their own worlds, or being unaware of body sensations. An *intrapersonal rhythm* might involve matching one's breath with one's movement (e.g., breathing in as one rolls the shoulders upward and exhaling when rolling downward). An *interpersonal rhythm* might involve matching one's movements with those of the group.

An additional valuable resource for both clinicians and trauma clients is van der Kolk's (2014) book *The Body Keeps the Score: Brain, Mind, and Body in the Healing of Trauma*, which focuses on the role of the body in processing trauma. It describes at considerable length the neurophysiology of trauma and how specific interventions, such as yoga, can be helpful in dealing with trauma. In yoga, a person focuses attention on their breathing and sensations from moment to moment. They begin to notice the connections between their emotions and body—perhaps how experiencing anxiety while doing a pose throws them off balance. They begin to experiment with changing the way they feel. Will taking a deep breath relieve that tension in their shoulder? Will focusing on their exhalations produce a sense of calm (van der Kolk, 2014, p. 273)? This resource gives one an appreciation of the reasoning behind why body interventions like yoga can be so helpful in treating trauma.

The body reactions to trauma are detailed in Peter Levine's (2010) book *In an Unspoken Voice*. Levine made the case that body interventions—yoga for example—are needed to treat trauma because trauma registers in a person's body far more than it does in other spheres, such as cognition, sensation, and perception. Levine described the condition of *fear paralysis* that is often seen in animals who have failed to escape a predator. Once they are caught, they often go into an unmoving state of paralysis. Levine reasoned that such immobility inhibits the aggressive instincts of the predator and perhaps confuses the attacker into seeing the victim as already dead. Some predators have little interest in prey that is already dead and show little inclination to attack further. Humans are presented as animals that react to trauma and life-threatening situations in the same way animals do because we are animals. Rape victims sometimes have great difficulty understanding why they did not fight their attacker more vigorously. It is possible that they are displaying the same fear paralysis seen in the animal kingdom. Immobility may be instinctually associated with survival. The focus of the bodily therapies advocated in Levine's book is intended to bring about a greater connection between body and mind that have been separated by traumatic experiences. Yoga can be an excellent tool to facilitate a reuniting of emotional and cognitive self with one's body. Trauma brings about separation. Yoga is a yoking of body and mind.

CASE EXAMPLE: EMILY'S SCHOOL REFUSAL

The case I'm about to describe shows that yoga can be of benefit not just to traumatized adults but also to children. Yoga sometimes results in surprising and unexpected benefits.

When I saw Emily a few years ago, she was an 11-year-old, highly verbal, and personable child who had a ready and beautiful smile for everyone she met. She was charming and bright by anyone's definition, the daughter any parent would love to have. All of this exterior positivity hid deep-seated feelings of worthlessness and painful, gnawing sensations associated with feeling unloved and unwanted. When required to go to school, she exhibited a barrage of ongoing physical complaints from colds, to body pains, to stomach problems. On school days, when she actually did attend, she would use a cane, limping down the hallway while holding her painful stomach.

Emily received a multitude of punishments for her school absences in the form of not being able to watch TV, no cell phone, and no friends over, but many of these punishments were unenforceable because her parents weren't home much. Emily's mother was a busy lawyer who arose early and did not return home until late. She insisted it was important for Emily to learn to fend for herself just like her own mother had done. It was Emily's responsibility to get up, get dressed, and make it to the bus stop. The refrigerator was stocked with food on weekends so that Emily would have food to eat during the week. A neglect complaint to Child Protective Services, perhaps initiated by a family member, had been filed but did not result in any enforceable action. Emily's father was a long-haul trucker who was home for two evenings once every 2 weeks. His relationship with Emily was remote, and the same could be said about his relationship with his wife. Emily's parents came across to me as tenants who lived in the same house, contributed to the bills, and viewed Emily as the burden that they both had to unwillingly bear. Emily was seen as, and clearly felt like, an afterthought to her parents.

When her mother brought Emily to me, she described Emily as ungrateful, whiney, never happy, and constantly complaining about imagined physical issues that kept her home from school. The contrast between the charming, bright, and chatty little girl I knew and the one her mother described was remarkable. Emily brought in coloring books and drawings she made. They were of good quality, and it was clear that she was seeking my praise and approval. She received plenty of both and seemed pleased. When our discussions turned to school attendance, Emily's face darkened, a wall went up, and she refused to discuss the matter. All she would say was, "They don't believe I don't feel well." Try as I might, Emily was unwilling to discuss anything having to do with school. Although it was apparent that her problems went way beyond school, I developed behavior management programs focusing on rewarding adaptive behavior, such as going to school and keeping things neat in the house. The rewards included playdates, going to McDonald's, and various toys and electronic games Emily were earned through a point system. My focus was not only on getting Emily to do what she was expected to do but also to get her parents to focus on Emily and her behavior, and to take a positive, rewarding stance to both.

My efforts to change Emily and her parent's behavior met with little to no success. I believe that in Emily's universe, being sick meant getting some consistent little bit of attention from her mother and from nurses, physicians, and psychologists. And then, one day, much to my amazement, Emily announced that she was going to school and looking forward to it. I practically fell out of my chair.

When I asked her what happened, she stated that the school had instituted a morning yoga class and that she loved it. She reported that yoga helped her to be more aware of her body and body sensations, and that she found this awareness to be particularly calming. Emily said that yoga made her feel at peace and gave her a sense of "being happy and whole." This report was both pleasing and sad: That yoga should be the best thing in a little girl's life is heartbreaking, but at least it is better than nothing.

Along with her participation in the yoga class came a greater willingness on Emily's part to discuss her unhappiness with her homelife, including the very sad comment that she wished she had never been born. Yoga seemed to be one of the few things she looked forward to. Emily's willingness to go to school resulted in an improvement in her relationship with her parents, but she continued to spend a great deal of time alone. Happily, her maternal grandparents began to play an increasingly prominent and nurturing role in Emily's life, and, in many ways, made up for the lack of emotional nurturance from her parents. Emily's accidental encounter with yoga and its presumed benefits appear to have started a chain reaction in which a reduction in her physical complaints elicited more positive responses from her mother and an increased willingness on the part of her grandparents to take a greater role in her care. One can only speculate as to whether Emily found yoga to be a needed distraction, whether yoga practice allowed her a deeper self-awareness, or whether poses and stretches actually helped to alleviate physical pains. By her own account, yoga seemed to produce a greater awareness of and control over her body, and she found both pleasing and calming. I no longer see Emily but have heard from her mother that she is doing well overall, despite occasional regressions into the domain of physical complaints.

Emily's newfound ability to express herself and attend school brightened her moods at home and enhanced her relationship with her mother. Also, the involvement of her grandparents did a great deal to offset a downward spiral toward which this young girl was heading. The serendipitous encounter with a school-based yoga program may have allowed Emily to get in better touch with herself and her feelings, and also served to teach me that the benefits of yoga might be applicable to children as well as adults. This is an important lesson for clinicians. The value of yoga has taken many of us traditionally trained clinicians by surprise. Yoga can be a valuable alternative treatment or adjunct to traditional treatment. It is certainly worth considering in those cases in which one seems to have encountered an impasse to forward movement.

WHAT IS THE LEVEL OF EMPIRICAL SUPPORT FOR YOGA AS AN INTERVENTION FOR PTSD?

In the world of clinical psychology, the randomized controlled trial (RCT) is the gold standard of research acceptability. In a typical RCT a comparatively large group of participants, PTSD sufferers, for example, are randomly assigned to a treatment group under investigation, another valid form of intervention, and a control group that does not receive an intervention. In the ideal RCT, multiple therapists are often used to combat the possibility that it was the particular characteristics of a given therapist that led to effects. Researchers use multiple investigative sites, psychometrically valid and reliable measures, and a carefully scripted form of intervention (to enhance treatment fidelity), and they often have a follow-up period to see whether and if the outcomes of the intervention hold up over time. So, now the question becomes: Has yoga proven itself a valid form of intervention for PTSD using a series of RCTs as the standard? The answer is both yes and no because there are not many RCT studies of yoga in the literature. However, some promising RCTs can be found. What are we to make of this?

One possibility for the comparative lack of RCT evidence for yoga is that it is not a valid form of intervention. The problem with this interpretation is that RCTs investigating yoga are not abundant because this type of research is resource heavy, is usually conducted in conjunction with universities and colleges, and is often funded by grants. Yoga is simply not the kind of acceptable academic topic that cognitive behavior therapy is. In a report entitled *Efficacy of Complementary and Alternative Medicine Therapies for Posttraumatic Stress Disorder* (Strauss, Coeytaux, McDuffie, & Williams, 2011), funded by Veterans Affairs, there were few acceptable RCT studies of yoga and, by unfortunate implication, a testament to the lack of efficacy of yoga. So, in addition to the possibility that the lack of RCT findings suggests that yoga is ineffective, we have another possibility, which is that yoga has not been fairly vetted to determine its efficacy because of the costliness of RCTs.

The bottom line is simply that yoga has not attained the status of eye-movement desensitization and reprocessing (EMDR) as a valid alternative therapy for PTSD, shaky as that status may be to mainstream academics and clinicians. Yoga is not considered to be an empirically supported treatment by such bodies as the American Psychological Association and the International Society for Traumatic Stress Studies. Nevertheless, trauma sufferers seek out yoga as an alternative to "traditional" therapies, and, if testimonial evidence is of any value, yoga is indeed a valid form of treatment.

What Do Actual Yoga Research Studies Show?

Although few RCT-type studies are available that examine the effectiveness of yoga in treating PTSD, one such study was carried out by van der Kolk et al. in 2014. It included 64 women with treatment-resistant PTSD and who had histories of prolonged trauma of an interpersonal nature, such as physical abuse, neglect, and domestic violence. Ten weeks of yoga classes with a frequency of one per week resulted in significant reductions in PTSD, depression, dissociation, and engagement in behaviors, such as self-injury, in comparison with an attention control group (a seminar on women's health). A follow-up study (Rhodes, Spinazzola, & van der Kolk, 2016) conducted 1½ years later included 49 of the original participants. Results indicated that group assignment was not a significant predictor of longer term outcome; however, frequency of continued yoga practice was associated with greater reductions in PTSD and depression, as well as a greater likelihood of a loss of the PTSD diagnosis. So, in summary, the original RCT and the follow-up study supported yoga as a useful treatment modality for PTSD, and its continued use was subsequently found to enhance yoga's benefits.

The lack of difference between yoga and a control condition noted in the Rhodes et al. (2016) follow-up study was also found in the RCT of veterans conducted by Reinhardt et al. (2018). In that study, 51 male and female participants who were veterans were initially recruited for a 10-week yoga intervention. High dropout rates resulted in only nine in the yoga group and six in the no-treatment, assessment-only control. Both yoga and control groups showed significant reductions in PTSD. When control participants were later provided with the yoga intervention, they demonstrated significant improvement in PTSD over their baseline scores. Although the Reinhardt et al. study might be considered a gold standard RCT-type study, the relatively small number of participants in the final analysis makes the drawing of conclusions difficult.

Again, we are confronted with this issue: Many of those who experience PTSD, veterans, in the case of the Reinhardt et al. (2018) study, are reluctant to participate in studies of any kind, even an intervention as nontrauma focused as yoga. Reinhardt et al. noted that prior studies showed dropout rates for yoga ranging from 7% to 32%; for general psychotherapies, 0% to 54%; and for cognitive behavior therapy, 68% (p. 104). Again, it seems that one of the major reasons for the comparatively low dropout rate for yoga as a PTSD intervention is that it is easier to tolerate regardless of its efficacy or effectiveness.

A meta-analysis was performed on 19 RCTs of complimentary therapies, such as yoga and meditation (Gallegos, Crean, Pigeon, & Heffner, 2017) and involved a total of 1,173 participants. (Meta-analyses combine the results of many studies to reach overall conclusions.) Results indicated that these alternative interventions consistently yielded small to medium effect sizes and that both participants and clinicians desired such alternative approaches. These results mean that alternative interventions have impact, but the results are not earthshaking. Actually, the same could be said for most forms of traditional treatments. Indeed, 80% of Veterans Affairs facilities offer some form of complementary therapy. The authors concluded that complementary interventions like yoga increase client choice, can often be done in groups, and do not necessarily require doctoral-level practitioners, and that these approaches are both of value and warrant further study. Simply stated, alternative therapies seem to be far more popular than traditional approaches, and they work.

How Responsive Are Veterans to Treatment?

At this point, I would like to relate a personal experience relevant to how willing, or more accurately, how unwilling, veterans are to accept therapy. In Chapter 2, the discussion of EMDR noted that the majority of veterans choose to avoid therapy for PTSD and especially therapies that force them to confront their trauma, such as prolonged exposure therapy and, to a lesser extent, EMDR. This has an all too familiar ring to me.

I returned home from a Vietnam in 1971 after having served in the U.S. Army's First Cavalry Division (helicopters, not horses). We deplaned from Vietnam at Fort Lewis in Washington State, and about 50 of us whose obligation to the military had been met were gathered into a room and provided with information on the process of separating from the army. One of the people to address us was a sergeant associated with a medical treatment unit. He informed us that the army was obligated to investigate and treat us for any medical or psychological condition associated with our tour in Vietnam, and that while being treated, we would still be considered to be assigned to, and part of, the U.S. Army. He then asked for a show of hands of anyone reporting a medical condition. Dead silence. Not a single hand was raised. He looked puzzled because the army was going to provide treatment at no expense to us. He then asked if anyone would like to report a psychological condition and made it clear that treatment would cost us nothing. The government would pay for our treatment no matter what the cost. Again, dead silence. No one was willing to report a condition that would obligate him or her in any way to continued participation in an army that had engaged in the hellish experience of the Vietnam War. So, when you read in the scientific literature that only a minority of veterans opts for treatment for PTSD, you can be sure that the size of that minority is likely to be grossly overstated. Avoidance is an ominous roadblock to any form of "treatment" for those who have been traumatized and especially those diagnosed with PTSD. It is for that reason that yoga and other alternatives to traditional psychotherapy have found a place in the hearts and minds of veterans and other traumatized individuals. In addition to data from RCTs, the testimonial evidence from those who have been traumatized is clearly supportive of yoga as a popular form of treatment.

SUMMARY

The use of yoga as an intervention for PTSD is not on the same level as such treatments as EMDR and many of the cognitive behavior therapy approaches as far as empirical validation is concerned. Nevertheless, some types of RCTs and meta-analyses do support its use for treating PTSD. It is considered to be a resource for treating psychological trauma by the U.S. Department Veterans Affairs and by many clinicians who treat civilian trauma. From that point of view, it is a valid alternative treatment approach for those who have been traumatized by both civilian and military experiences.

4

Mindfulness Meditation-Based Interventions for PTSD

The term *meditation* arises from the Latin *meditatum*, which means to ponder (Mead, 2020). *Mindfulness* is an English translation of the word *sati*, which in the Pali language used by Buddhists 2,500 years ago implies attention, remembering, and awareness (Germer, Siegel, & Fulton, 2013, p. 5). Meditation has a long history, and some have placed its origins as many as 5,000 years ago (Dienstmann, 2018). It has been suggested that meditation may have arisen even earlier during times when cave dwellers experienced altered states of consciousness as they endured long hours in dark caves or perhaps spent time staring into the flames of comforting fires that provided warmth and security. The Hindus initiated the development of meditation as a way of getting closer to the true nature of God. Siddhartha Gautama, The Buddha, was said to have attained enlightenment around 500 BC and used meditation to better understand the relatedness of all things; thus, Buddhist practices focused more on this goal than on grasping the nature of God. A community of Japanese monks emphasized Zazen, or sitting meditation, during the eighth century; they focused on the interconnectedness of all things, animate and inanimate (Dienstmann, 2018).

Islam, Judaism, Christianity, Jainism, Sikhism, Taoism, Sufism, Native American, and other traditions all have their own forms of meditation and contemplative practices. Jewish meditative traditions include Kabbalah practices. Kabbalah seeks to delineate the nature of the universe and human beings, nature and purpose of existence, and other basic questions. Islamic meditation includes the repetition of God's name numerous times along with breathing

http://dx.doi.org/10.1037/0000186-005
Alternative Therapies for PTSD: The Science of Mind–Body Treatments, by R. W. Motta

controls to foster greater awareness (Ginsburgh, 2006). In Christian meditation, people repeat certain postures and prayers, and may use the rosary, which involves repeating prayers to foster greater awareness, spiritual purity, and closeness to God. Trappists are members of a Christian religious order of cloistered contemplative monastics that discourages idle speech. The resulting silence inhibits the temptation to exercise one's own will and fosters a meditation on, and awareness of, the will of God. Despite the connection between meditation and religion, the forms of meditation popular in the West today are not associated with any particular religion but instead emphasize awareness and acceptance of oneself, acceptance of others, the nature of one's current experiences, and an immersion in and appreciation of the present moment (Nisbet, 2017).

OVERVIEW OF MINDFULNESS-BASED MEDITATION

The awareness that evolves from meditation can eventuate in a greater self-knowledge and a far less critical and negative view of oneself and others. This nonjudgmental awareness includes the realization of and focus on the present moment. Focusing on the present, though, is a particularly problematic issue for those with posttraumatic stress disorder (PTSD) because their focus is primarily on their past and the terror of traumatizing experiences. The practice of meditation eventuates in an increasing liberation from the tyranny of one's ongoing stream of thought, or *stream of consciousness* to use a term attributed to William James (Editors of *Encyclopaedia Britannica*, n.d.). This stream of consciousness marches on constantly and seemingly independently of the wishes of the thinker. In general, meditation has two types: directive and nondirective. *Nondirective meditation* is a relaxed state of attention, and one simply observes spontaneously occurring thoughts, images, memories, emotions, and sensations. They do not attempt to stop these mind wanderings but simply observe them, note what they are, and let go of them. In *directive meditation*, one usually focuses on a particular activity or object. The most common object of attention in directive meditation is breathing. So, in this case, one would attend to the passage of air coming in and out of the body, and to the movement of upper parts of the body in response to breathing. When the mind wanders off to some thought, feeling, or sensation, the person pulls it back in to return the focus to breathing. Both forms of meditation emphasize nonjudgmental awareness and create a moving away from preoccupation of, and confinement by one's wandering thoughts. It is advisable to allow PTSD sufferers to choose which form of medication they would like to practice rather than suggest one form or the other. As previously noted in the material on yoga (see Chapter 3, this volume), choice is critically important among those whose freedom to choose was not an option during their traumatic experiences.

In practicing meditation, mind wanderings are increasingly replaced by being in the present moment and not being continuingly distracted by and led around by seemingly random thoughts. Typically, the untrained mind hops from one thought to another through a process of association. In many ways, the mind has a mind of its own, moving as it does from one thought to the next with little input from the thinker. The default mode network (e.g., Horn, Ostwald, Reisert, & Blankenburg, 2014) of the brain is active when one is engaged in nonfocused mental activity, such as mind wandering, an envisioning of the future and past, or whatever automatically occupies ones thoughts when they make no effort to focus their attention on a particular issue or concern. Key structural regions of this network that appear on brain scans are the medial prefrontal cortex and posterior cingulate cortex, and these areas are interconnected with the amygdala, which is associated with fear and fear conditioning. So, what this means is that most of time, when one is not engaged in focused attention, the mind wanders to thoughts of self, threats to self, and consequent emotional reactions to these threats:

> Studies have shown that these places [mind wanderings] are usually in the past or the future; you may ponder recent events or distant, strong memories; you may dread upcoming events or eagerly anticipate them. . . . What you're generally *not* doing when your mind is wandering is directly experiencing the present moment. (Wright, 2017, p. 46)

With meditative practice, one develops increasingly focused attention, less thought distraction, and a weakening of the apprehensions resulting from connections between the medial prefrontal cortex, posterior cingulate cortex, and amygdala. These explanations may be well and good, yet a conceptualization of mindfulness is not easily put into words, as Germer (2005) pointed out: "Mindfulness has to be experienced to be known" (p. 8). It is a subtle, nonverbal experience (Gunaratana, 2002). One cannot actually grasp love without having experienced it, and it might be that this necessity of experience is also true of mindfulness to grasp its true meaning:

> We tend to be particularly unaware that we are thinking virtually all the time. The incessant stream of thoughts flowing through our minds leaves us very little respite for inner quiet. . . . Meditation means learning how to get out of this current, sit by the bank and listen to it, learn from it, and then use its energies to guide us rather than to tyrannize us. (Kabat-Zinn, 1994, p. 9)

In addition to the novelty of freeing oneself from the ongoing stream of thought, it is important to consider another novel issue: one's objectives in practicing mindfulness. The goal of meditation practice may be at odds with traditional therapies, such as cognitive behavior therapy (CBT). Whereas traditional therapeutic approaches seek symptom reduction and objective, replicable procedures, meditation teaches that symptoms are transitory phenomena and outcomes of meditation are unique to the individual, so, in that way, are subjective. In mindfulness practice, one is to observe, accept, and understand symptoms, and not necessarily react to or intentionally alter or reduce those symptoms. In meditating, psychological well-being comes from reducing the struggle against symptoms, accepting them, and finding peace and gratitude in the current moment and learning to live in the now. This stance is clearly at odds with traditional medically influenced views of CBT that emphasize the primacy of symptom reduction and replicable methods.

BRIEF HISTORY OF MINDFULNESS IN THERAPY

The adaptation of mindfulness for treating PTSD is a recent development, probably most often taken up by returning combatants from the wars in Iraq and Afghanistan. Trauma-sensitive mindfulness practice has been written about only within the past few years (Treleaven, 2018). Although mindfulness practices may date back thousands of years, their relationship to psychotherapy and psychotherapists may be traced back to era of Freud (1930/1961), who wrote of an oceanic feeling experienced in meditation but nevertheless saw meditation as a regressive experience. Many other well-known clinicians and writers such as Erich Fromm, Karen Horney, Carl Jung, and others wrote about and triggered an interest in Buddhism and Eastern views. During the 1960s, the Beatles and other famous individuals and groups went on pilgrimages to India and began to popularize mindfulness and Eastern philosophies, which served to stoke the embers of therapeutic interest. The book *Be Here Now* by Harvard University psychologist and former professor Ram Dass (1971), who was born Richard Alpert in a prominent Massachusetts family, was a popular bestseller on mindfulness; sales have reached more than 2 million copies ("A Brief Organizational History," n.d.). He had traveled to India to learn more about methods of attaining greater awareness; previously, he had relied on hallucinogenic drugs for inspiration and had encouraged others to do so. This involvement of students in taking drugs is reportedly what cost him his job as a professor.

In 1975, Herbert Benson's book *The Relaxation Response* detailed breathing and other mindfulness practices, which led to physical and psychological health benefits. Benson, a cardiologist, pointed out a link between cardiac disease and stress, as well as the benefits that accrue through regular meditative practice. A major figure in popularizing mindfulness in the United States has been Jon Kabat-Zinn. Philip Kapleau, a Zen missionary, introduced Kabat-Zinn to meditation while Kabat-Zinn was working toward a doctorate in molecular biology at the Massachusetts Institute of Technology. Kabat-Zinn went on to study with other meditation teachers, including Thich Nhat Hanh. In 1979, Kabat-Zinn founded the Stress Reduction Clinic at the University of Massachusetts Medical School; there, he adapted the Buddhist teaching of mindfulness and created the stress reduction and relaxation program ("Jon Kabat-Zinn," n.d.). The clinic emphasized mindfulness-based stress reduction (MBSR), which was an 8-week intensive program teaching mindfulness practices and was open to those suffering from various chronic and terminal diseases, and others in psychological distress. The MBSR clients and staff practiced meditation 45 minutes a day for the 8-week period in addition to other health-oriented initiatives. Kabat-Zinn subsequently founded the Center for Mindfulness in Medicine, Health Care, and Society at the University of

Massachusetts Medical School, and this center teaches clients how to deal with pain, stress, illness, and disease through the practice of mindfulness (Center for Mindfulness in Medicine, Health Care, and Society, n.d.).

Kabat-Zinn later began to draw increasing attention with his books *Full Catastrophe Living: Using the Wisdom of Your Body and Mind to Face Stress, Pain, and Illness* (1990); *Wherever You Go, There You Are: Mindfulness Meditation in Everyday Life* (1994); and *Coming to Our Senses: Healing Ourselves and the World Through Mindfulness* (2005). The publication of a mindfulness-based treatment approach for depression and depressive relapse (Teasdale et al., 2000) contributed to awareness that mindfulness has an empirically supported place in cognitively based psychotherapy. Langer's (2014) book *Mindfulness: 25th Anniversary Edition* provided numerous experiments and practical examples of the benefits of mindful states.

To a large extent, mindfulness has gone mainstream. It is an exceedingly popular topic for books, articles, and other forms of academic and social media. This explosion of interest is further reflected in the number of therapeutic approaches, such as dialectical behavior therapy (Linehan, 1993) and acceptance and commitment therapy (Hayes, Strosahl, & Wilson, 2016), that have incorporated mindfulness practices as an important component of their decidedly CBT framework. Therefore, mindfulness may be viewed as an important component of empirically validated practice (Hayes, Follette, & Linehan, 2004).

WHAT IS MINDFULNESS?

One would think that with such an exponential growth of interest in mindfulness that the concept could be clearly defined and the techniques to attain mindful awareness would be specifically delineated. That is not the case. Many different practices and definitions exist. According to Kabat-Zinn (1994), "Mindfulness means paying attention in particular way: on purpose, in the present moment, and non-judgmentally" (p. 4). In his MBSR training program previously mentioned ("Jon Kabat-Zinn," n.d.), one could achieve mindfulness through the process of sitting, standing, lying down, walking, eating, and doing yoga exercises. What this process suggests is that there is no "best" way to attempt to develop mindfulness; it can occur through various activities. A person can practice mindfulness while driving, emptying the dishwasher, mowing the lawn, doing the laundry, or engaging in just about any activity common to human beings. According to Germer (2005), what mindfulness practices have in common are awareness, a focus on present experience, and (nonjudgmental) acceptance.

Awareness

Awareness often, although not necessarily, entails the cessation of automatic semiconscious activity and a focus on what is taking place now. It is particularly relevant for the PTSD sufferer who is so preoccupied with their past, that awareness of the present often fades into insignificance. So, for example, one could stop reading their e-mail or obsessing about the past and sit on a cushion or chair and focus on their feelings and sensations associated with sitting or focus on the process of breathing. The practitioner in this case might focus on the air passing through the nostrils or the expansion and contraction of the chest area and diaphragm, or the feeling of support at the underside of the legs. Alternatively, one could continue a common activity, such as walking, but do it far more slowly, noticing what area of the foot touches the ground first, what foot area then follows, how the weight shifts from one side of the body to the next in readiness for the other foot to make contact, and how this process creates movement and change in sensations. "Awareness is not the same as thought," said Kabat-Zinn (1994). "It lies beyond thinking. . . . Awareness is more like a vessel which can hold and contain our thoughts as thoughts rather than getting caught up in them as reality" (p. 93). What Kabat-Zinn seems to suggest is that awareness involves knowing what is presently taking place, including the content of one's thoughts without viewing these thoughts as representing reality. Our thoughts represent our concerns and interests. They are self-created and are not reality. Indeed, we may be living in an unreal dream world comprising our thinking. Perhaps a goal of mindfulness is an appreciation of what is real and what is self-created or illusory. In mindfulness meditation, one observes what thoughts pass through one's mind but does not pursue them.

Focus on Present Activity

Often ongoing thought presents itself as ruminations. For example, those with PTSD may mentally rehearse prior intensely negative encounters. They may replay conversations that they had or reenact interpersonal situations in which they might have acted differently. Perhaps those with PTSD are ruminating on some future activities or events that are in the works. Mental activity usually involves ruminations regarding the past or the future, but far less often, is it in the present. During mindfulness meditation, one attempts to observe present activity, and traditionally this activity involves observation of the process of breathing, although it need not do so. One can also focus on bodily sensations, sounds in the environment, temperature changes, odors, or anything else that is currently—and that is the critical word—taking place.

What invariably happens during meditation is that thoughts arise, and these thoughts are often part of the ongoing stream of ruminations of past and present preoccupations. In practicing mindfulness, one simply notes what the thought is and thereby learns what their preoccupations are, and then one returns to an awareness of the present moment by breathing, for example.

The process just described results in a self-knowledge, a nonjudgmental understanding and self-awareness. Some practitioners of mindfulness meditation (e.g., "How to Begin Naming," n.d.) have suggested that whatever arises during, for example, a focus on breathing, label it (e.g., "a fear," "a want," "a worry") and then return to an awareness of breathing. With repeated practice, one begins to develop an increasing capability to be aware of what is happening in the present moment. So, for example, when eating, one is aware of taste sensations, texture, chewing, the formation of saliva, and swallowing. Contrast this awareness with what happens more frequently when people eat: They hardly or only briefly notice the food while their mind wanders to other issues. While dressing for work, a person may be only momentarily aware what clothes they are putting on, but their mind is focused on planning the activities of the day, people they will encounter, or problems they must solve. Rarely is the focus on colors, textures, alignment, or the feel of one's clothing, and if it is on one of these things, it only occupies only a small amount of time. With continued meditative practice, one becomes increasingly aware of what normally flits by one's awareness, and in doing so, that person is simply and wonderfully present.

Nonjudgment

This aspect of mindfulness is alternatively called acceptance. When meditating, it is not uncommon to make judgments, such as "I'm doing better at this [or I am not] than I used to," "What's wrong with me? Why can't I stay focused on the present?" or, for those suffering with prior trauma, "I can't believe I let that happen to me" or "I acted like an animal in that situation." Rather than engaging in negative self-assessments, one accepts the present experience of one's meditation without evaluative judgment. Similarly, one accepts without evaluation the nagging tendency of ruminations and preoccupations to interfere with one's meditation. It is best to accept that intrusions will occur thousands of times during one's meditations, that this is normal, and that with each intrusion, to return to the breath or other chosen focus of attention. Thought intrusion and preoccupation are seen simply as activities of the mind. and the same can be said for one's symptoms. They are not judged as good or bad but simply accepted as being.

Unfortunately, just like ruminations and preoccupations, the process of judgment rarely stops, or if it does, it is not for long. People will even judge that they are judging: "When will I learn to stop being so judgmental?" is a negative evaluation of one's tendency to evaluate. These aspects of meditation—being aware, present, and nonjudgmental—are outcomes of meditation practice, and one frequently engages in this practice for years. In mindfulness meditation, one strives for awareness, presence of mind, and a nonevaluative stance and an acceptance that these are lifelong quests. As such, mindfulness is not like eye-movement desensitization and reprocessing (EMDR), acceptance and commitment therapy, or dialectical behavior therapy—the latter two include a mindfulness component—which are interventions to reduce symptoms. Once a person achieves their therapeutic objectives, they no longer need EMDR, acceptance and commitment therapy, or dialectical behavior therapy.

Mindfulness is more of a stance that one develops over a lifetime. It may be best to consider meditation practice a lifelong endeavor like healthy eating and exercise. It is not an intervention per se.

MECHANICS OF MINDFULNESS

Questions often arise about how one can actually get started practicing mindfulness. The material to follow addresses the setting, amount of time to practice, body positions, and other specific issues. The importance of regular daily practice cannot be overemphasized in achieving the benefits of mindfulness.

Setting and Position

Whether one suffers from PTSD or not, it is best to have a specific place where one practices because it will contribute to the formation of a habit. I discuss specific meditative approaches for PTSD in a later section. In general, this place should be relatively free of distractions and intrusions. By having a specific place, it is more likely that one will establish a habit of location and time of meditation practice. One might choose to have a *zafu*, that is, a meditation cushion on which to sit, or a straight-backed chair; may simply walk slowly and attentively in a common place; or may lie down in *savasana*, also called the corpse pose. This pose involves being on one's back, feet about hip width apart, palms facing upward and spaced slightly away from the body, and eyes usually closed. It's not often a good idea, though, to practice meditation in bed because it will foster falling asleep.

Most forms of meditation involve sitting in a particular place. If one is sitting on a straight-backed chair, it is a good idea to sit with an erect, dignified posture such that the back is not touching the back of the chair. If sitting on a cushion, sit with an erect posture, which fosters alertness and attention. When thoughts intrude and one begins to follow them, they tend to lose the erect posture and their shoulders sag. The goal is to then observe the content of the thought; return to a focus on, say, breathing; and resume the erect posture. Although it is good practice to establish a routine of meditation practice, mindfulness can take place anywhere while engaging in most activities. While standing and looking outside, for example, one observes the trees and the movement of the leaves with the wind, the birds, the tree branches, and the feeling of the floor beneath one's feet, all without evaluation and without judgments like good or bad.

Time

What is the best time to meditate? How long does one meditate? The first question seems somewhat answerable; the second, less so. Most writers (e.g., Harris & Warren, 2017) suggest meditating in the morning. One's living space is usually quiet in the morning, and practicing early sets the tone for the day, one of awareness and attentiveness. Also, it is easy to find innumerable important reasons for other matters to take priority over meditating when pushing the practice to later in the day: "I forgot to return Mary's email," "I must remember to pay the bills," or "I just can't leave those unwashed dishes in the sink." By practicing in the morning, it is almost as if one is giving mindfulness practice priority over just about anything else that needs doing. The longer a person waits to meditate, the far more likely they will recall something that they must do (e.g., "Time is passing. I have to get this done!"). Practicing early in the morning is the ideal, and yet it may not be possible or even desirable for everyone. If it can't be done, simply accept it and try to practice at a more reasonable and available time. Again, the establishment of an early morning routine is desirable for the reasons stated previously and also because one is more attentive and less fatigued during the early part of the day. Nevertheless, some people simply are not "morning people," and for them, practice at a later time may be valuable. What is important is that meditative practice be done regularly.

Kabat-Zinn (1994) stated that the question of how much time to spend meditating often comes up, and his response is as follows: "How should I know?" (p. 121). In his MBSR program at the University of Massachusetts, the routine was 45 minutes every day for 8 weeks. However, he claimed that if all you have is 5 minutes, that is fine; the sincerity and focus of the practice are what is important. If one is new to the practice of meditation, perhaps starting with brief amounts of time is best, and then progressively building up the time with further sessions is a good idea. In a study of more than 600 individuals, Soler et al. (2014) found that frequency of mindfulness practice and lifetime experience practicing mindfulness were associated with self-reported mindfulness but that length of time during each session was not. They recommended meditating 20 minutes a day, and this length is a commonly suggested one. A degree of individual variation exists, however. Some people are able to settle the mind into a meditative state more quickly than others. Those who do not settle quickly may require more time to quiet the incessant chatter of thoughts. If one has low frustration tolerance, is anxious, has many demands on their time, or tends to be overly judgmental, it might be best to start with shorter periods of practice and then build up slowly. A reasonable response to the question, How long should I meditate? is that regularity of practice seems more important than session length. It is somewhat like the question, What is the best relaxation technique? The best technique is the one the person finds they are most likely to repeat. So, if one meditates for an amount of time that they can handle, that will encourage them to keep practicing.

Posture

One can practice mindfulness while sitting, walking, lying down, or being engaged in just about any activity, as mentioned earlier, but probably the most common and recognizable form of practice is sitting meditation. Sit erect in a dignified posture on a cushion or on a straight-backed chair. If on a chair, it is advisable to sit away from the back of the chair. Posture is important because it aids in developing concentration, focus, and alertness.

Sometimes these erect postures are not as comfortable as resting against the back of the chair or slumping. The mild discomfort of sitting erect can itself become a focus of one's meditation: One may see that handling discomfort and facing it might also aid in helping them to confront and deal with other discomforts, such as emotional pain. When noticing that one's posture is not what it "should" be, the person is making a judgment, and awareness of this judgment facilitates the inclination to developing a nonjudging, accepting stance. So, rather than criticize oneself for not having an erect posture, it is more in keeping with the attitude of nonjudging to accept that one has lost their erect posture, and this is a common occurrence. One corrects their posture and realizes that their focus has drifted to posture. They return their attention to focusing on breathing or another focus of the meditation. Oddly, what one is developing is awareness of awareness. With practice, one becomes increasingly attuned to where their awareness drifts. In the case of our awareness drifting to posture, posture is both a component of mindfulness and a target of their awareness.

Sequence

As indicated earlier, methods of practicing mindfulness abound, many of which involve stillness and some that involve movement. However, based on my clinical experience, the sequence looks like the following:

1. Establish a comfortable and attentive position whether sitting, standing, or lying down. If sitting, the goal is to sit erect in a dignified attentive posture. If lying down, try to be aware of the floor or mat supporting the length of your body and have your arms and legs slightly away from the body.

2. Close your eyes or look downward at a place 2 or 3 feet in front of you. If your eyes are open, it is not necessary to maintain a clear focus on an object or thing because, ultimately, your focus is within. Typically, a person's eyes are either closed or half closed but are not necessarily focused.

3. Pay attention to your breathing by perhaps paying attention to the air passing through the nostrils and throat or the slow up-and-down movement of the chest and abdomen.

4. Attempt to maintain this attention, but when thoughts intrude, as they invariably will, note the content of the thought and return your attention to the breathing. Accept that it is normal and expected to have unwanted thoughts interrupt your focus, and that being aware of the moment when this happens is a component of mindfulness.

5. Once you are able to focus on the breathing, you might include other areas of attention. For example, you can focus on the sensations of the body,

whether they are comfortable or uncomfortable, all while taking the stance of the nonjudgmental observer. You might listen to the sound of traffic or movement within your home. You might even focus on odors or temperature sensations.

6. Become aware of the reasons why you are eventually ending the session. Do you feel it has been long enough? Are you impatient? Is there something you feel the need to attend to? Knowing the reasons becomes part of the process of developing nonjudgmental awareness.

7. Practice, practice, practice.

SPECIFIC MINDFULNESS PRACTICES FOR TRAUMA AND PTSD

Let's recall that one of the critical factors in the development of PTSD is confinement and lack of choice. Those who develop PTSD often find themselves in situations involving extreme threat and overwhelming fear coupled with an inability to escape them. When one has the ability to escape, they are able to exercise control and have a lessened likelihood of developing PTSD. For this reason, it is important that meditative practice for trauma and PTSD should be flexible in its methods and that the person doing the meditation should not feel confined in any way.

This emphasis on freedom and choice starts with the location and time of meditative practice. The traumatized person should be able select a place in which they feel secure. So, for example, one's own living space may be far more desirable than a mediation hall where others surround the traumatized person. The person should have the freedom to change the location and the time when the meditation takes place. Choice is critical. One can choose to pay attention to their thoughts, feelings, and sensations, but in the beginning, this may be too much to handle. Traumatized individuals often feel overwhelmed by crushing body sensations (van der Kolk, 2014) painful memories, and extremes of anxiety. Although it is common for mindfulness meditation to focus on the present flow of thoughts, images, and sensations, it might be less threatening for the trauma victim to initially focus on far more neutral stimuli. For instance, one may wish to focus on a spot on the floor a few feet away or engage in breath counting. Here, the practitioner might count breaths one through five and then reverse, five to one, and continue this pattern for whatever period they like. The trauma victim might then choose to gently touch on experiences that were traumatic or to do so only briefly and then return to a focus on the breath or on self-compassion. If a trusted clinician is administering the mindfulness meditation, it is crucial to present the various practices in a nondirective manner that emphasizes client freedom of choice.

Trauma victims often have problems with concentration and focus, and emotional arousal heightens these problems. This difficulty with concentration may be an unconscious safety-enhancing process that tones down the clarity and pain of traumatic memories. When these memories become overwhelming, the trauma victim may experience *dissociation* in which they blank out on trauma memories and images, as well as disconnect from them. *Flashbacks* are common and involve unwanted intrusive images, sensations, and memories of the traumatic event; they also can trigger dissociation. The trauma victim may experience *depersonalization* whereby they are suddenly uncertain who they are and how they fit into the current environment. *Derealization* may occur; in this case, the victim feels that their present environment is surreal, unrecognizable, and thereby anxiety provoking. Again, all of these processes may represent unconscious attempts by the mind to protect the victim from something that is overwhelming and impossible to tolerate.

Clearly, clinicians working the those who have PTSD must move forward with great sensitivity, patience, and awareness of the overwhelming nature of this disorder. In the beginning of treatment, it is important to establish parameters to ensure that the client is in no way emotionally overwhelmed. Doing so can be truly difficult to accomplish because many trauma survivors are so easily overtaken by just about anything that brings up painful memories and images. Trauma treatment, whether it is mindfulness oriented or comes in some other form, often demands a great deal from clinicians. A good deal of research shows that therapists and anyone else having close and extended contact with trauma victims often begin to show trauma symptoms themselves (e.g., McCann & Pearlman, 1990; Motta, 2013). With recovery from trauma comes increasing empowerment and choice (Turow, 2017), and a lessened emotional response to trauma stimuli.

In many cases, trauma treatment must go at a slow pace so that the client is able to tolerate the treatment. It is also important for clinicians to not push those with PTSD to meditate for a given amount of time; instead, clinicians need to flexible and sensitive to the possible need for the client to slowly increase the time that they engage in meditation. The medical model of treatment that has impacted much of psychological and psychiatric interventions is that disorders must be overcome quickly and efficiently. This mantra of quickly and efficiently solving problems is not applicable to the grief that one experiences in losing a loved one. This book reflects my recognition that individuals make adjustments at a pace they can tolerate. It might be helpful for clinicians to develop the same view when treating trauma, whether using mindfulness or some other method. The clinician must permit, allow, and even encourage their clients to move forward at a tempo they can tolerate, even when this pace seems painfully slow to that clinician.

Mountain Meditation

Because it emphasizes strength and endurance, *mountain meditation* can be helpful for those who have experienced trauma and PTSD. Traumatized individuals may be so severely shaken by their overwhelming experiences that they often do not recognize the person they have become and feel vulnerable in, and suspicious of, their environment. For most of us, we can put life difficulties into a context that can "make sense," and thus we continue to feel that life events are predictable and understandable. Victims suffering from PTSD may have encountered situations that are so overwhelming that they don't make sense, and they have difficulty putting those situations into any understandable context. In addition, the PTSD sufferer sees themselves acting in ways reminiscent of how a frightened animal might respond following traumatic experiences. Having seen themselves respond in this way, they begin to doubt that their original self-perception was reality based or whether this new anxiety-laden self is an accurate representation of who they are. Thus, not only is the environment alien and threatening to the trauma victim but their very sense of self might also be something they find strange. It is not far from the truth to say that a trauma victim becomes a *Stranger in a Strange Land*, to borrow the title from a well-known science fiction book (Heinlein, 1961).

The mountain meditation can be a useful first step in helping those who have been traumatized because rather than focusing on awareness of sensations and feelings, it emphasizes solidity, strength, and endurance. This form of meditation can be helpful to those whose lives, sense of self, and perceptions of safety and predictability have been called into question. The assurance of safety and security should be the basis of any form of therapeutic intervention, and the same is true in this meditation. One should not venture into self-exploration when the sense of self is unstable and the person holds a view of an unpredictable environment.

The meditation is usually done in a sitting posture. One directs their attention to the characteristics of a mountain. The mountain endures the environmental changes of temperature, wind, rain, tourists, and everything else. People and other living creatures go about their daily lives and change in time, whereas plants grow, waves crash upon the shore, and rivers rush or run dry, yet the mountain remains relatively unchanged, solid, and unaffected. Snow may accumulate on its peak and rivulets may pour down its sides during heavy rains, but at the end of the day, the mountain remains relatively unscathed and unchanged.

During the mountain meditation, one's legs and buttocks may be seen as the base of the mountain: stable and unmoving. The head is envisioned as the top of the mountain: buffeted by wind, covered by snow, and dampened by rain but unfazed and unchanged. The shoulders and arms may represent the sides of the mountain and its features. The enduring solidity of the mountain is mindfully viewed as one with the self. Thus, one sees the self as solid, unmoved, unflinching, and enduring. These perceptions can bring a real sense of relief and anxiety reduction to the trauma and PTSD sufferer, and can be a valuable first step in the healing process. The mountain meditation provides much needed stability and tranquility. It is a wonderful first step for trauma victims who must make a long and difficult journey, and will ultimately lead to the discovery or rediscovery of who they are and their relationship to others and to the environment.

Lake Meditation

The *lake meditation* is capable of bringing a sense of tranquility and peace to those suffering the emotional storms created by traumatic experiences. It is often done lying down or in a sitting posture. One envisions a clear and placid lake, which may be occasionally roiled by wind and rain but ultimately returns to its tranquil self once these disturbances have passed. During meditation, one imagines the lake and its various characteristics in detail. With focused practice, a oneness with the nature of the lake and water takes place. The lake "is cradled in a receptive basin by the earth itself" (Kabat-Zinn, 1994, p. 141) and forms part of the tranquil, calm-promoting environment. The lake is receptive to those who wish to boat on it and, in many ways, is even more unmoved and enduring than the mountain. Regardless of the disturbances that it endures, it returns to its placid self. The lake cannot be permanently impacted or changed. It can be penetrated but returns to its still self and remains unchanged. It comprises one of the basic elements of earth and is life giving and life sustaining. The lake is both tranquil and enduring. It is for these reasons that the lake meditation can be a good follow-up to the mountain meditation. Solidity and tranquility are characteristics much needed by those who have been altered by traumatic experience.

Clinicians can consider the lake and mountain meditations to be useful first steps along the way to healing from trauma. These meditations do not demand that the victim confront and deal with their emotional damage or their memories of what happened to them. Such confrontations and the overwhelming pain that they induce are the very reasons why trauma victims avoid therapy. In place of such confrontations, these two meditations present visions of tranquility, stability, evenness, and predictability, all of which are lacking in the lives of trauma survivors. The meditations are wonderful first steps that, from the clinician's perspective, are designed to build up and strengthen the trauma survivor so that growth and healing can occur.

Loving-Kindness Meditation

Once the PTSD or trauma victim has attained some level of stability through the initial meditative steps of the mountain and lake meditations, the clinician can consider the loving-kindness meditation. *Consideration* is the crucial word because initiating this meditation requires clinical judgment and sensitivity. Recall that trauma survivors are often alienated from themselves and have a wary, suspicious view of their environment. The *loving-kindness meditation* initially involves a focus of love and caring toward oneself. But what if one is uncertain about who they are? Do they continue feel dehumanized owing to a rape, or physical abuse, or other extremely frightening violation of self? If so, engaging in a meditation that requires having a stable and at least partially worthy sense of self might not only be extremely difficult but highly troubling and potentially damaging. If the trauma victim has attained a level of stability and recovery such that they are beginning to recover and reinhabit much of what they once were, then this meditation might be beneficial. If not, please be cautious. Many clients have fled the well-intended efforts of caring clinicians because they became overwhelmed and were unable deal with what their clinician presented.

Once one is centered and has attained a tranquil and a quiet mind state, the practice begins with an expanding and evolving intention toward goodwill. During the meditation, one silently repeats certain phrases to themselves (Salzberg, 1995), such as "May I be safe. May I be happy. May I have peace. May I be healthy. May I have tranquility. May my actions be kind." Again, acceptance of these phrases may not come easily to those with a prior history of trauma, abuse, or neglect. These kinds of experiences breed a sense or low self-worth and lack of deservingness. The positive phrases should be repeated, and when intruding thoughts come in because of the potential discomfort that they may induce, the unwanted thought is supplanted by further repetitions of the phrases. When one begins to accept their deservingness of love (and this might take a long time), their value as a caring human being, and their dignity and worth, they might want to wade in the warm pool of this love and acceptance, and then stay there and become part of the loving warmth emanating from the very heart of kindness and love. There is no essential need to move further, but because we are all interconnected and share similar wants, desires, and concerns, a felt need may arise to spread the loving-kindness outward to include others.

Moving outward, one might wish to spread the beliefs of deservingness of love and care to siblings, children, and parents who are living or dead. Love them and forgive them for any pains they may have caused the sufferer or others. Realize that those who have been pained most often cause pain. The focus of mindfulness can then grow to include loving-kindness that the client spreads to acquaintances, colleagues, coworkers, and friends. With time and practice, they can spread these feelings of goodwill to others, to those who live in other neighborhoods, to those in other lands. Those whom one dislikes and those whose behaviors one finds repugnant might also become recipients of their mindful good will and positive intentions. The client may be inclined to wish benefits and goodwill to pets, other nonhuman organisms, and to our breathing, living planet. In doing so, they are, as Kabat-Zinn (1994) put it, stretching "against the boundaries . . . of [their] minds and hearts" or are stating, as Kabat-Zinn quoted the Dalai Lama, "My religion is kindness" (p. 168). The client's sharing of kindness and love to others becomes an enhancing process of love of themselves once they have accepted the interconnectedness of all things.

Alas, few things of value are easily obtained. Meditation is certainly useful, particularly for those suffering from PTSD, but it does require concerted effort and discipline. It is difficult to obtain statistics on those who meditate, but it is highly likely that the majority of those who begin meditating eventually stop because of the effort required to maintain an ongoing practice over extended periods and perhaps a lifetime. Many have speculated that the human brain, with its approximately 90 billion interconnected neurons, is primarily not conscious and that only a small part of the brain's activity rises to the level awareness. Damasio (2010) speculated that the brain contains modules, such as one for recent experience, past experience, desires, wants, needs, and interpersonal interactions, and these modules compete for a place on the stage of awareness. If a module is not given attention, as is likely to happen when one meditates, another may take its place. This perpetual competition for a place on the awareness stage is experienced as a stream of intruding thoughts when one meditates. Not following thoughts that have arisen during meditation practice is an ongoing process even for experienced meditators, and the effort involved will often deter many who may wish to attempt meditation over a long period. PTSD victims and those who simply wish to obtain a greater awareness can derive significant benefits from meditation, and these benefits require sustained, focused practice.

CASE EXAMPLE: COPING WITH TRAUMA FROM UNINTENDED HARM

Susan was raised by parents who believed in hard work, discipline, and adherence to the word of God. Before a troubling series of events that I describe shortly, Susan was a strong-willed child who took a certain pleasure in pushing whatever limits were set for her; overall, though, she was well behaved, was not a problem child, and did well in school. As a 58-year-old, she presented herself in therapy as a highly anxious, disheveled, and generally not well-groomed elementary school teacher. On probing the roots of her difficulties, it came to light that they seem to have come about when she was in kindergarten. It was around the time of Halloween, and children were required to draw and color pumpkins. The nuns at her Catholic girls' school were quite strict and insisted that the students draw pumpkins of certain sizes and color them orange. Susan, as was typical of her pleasant though mischievous nature, drew her pumpkin with precision but, once again testing the limits, colored it green. The strict nun who taught this class not only did not appreciate what she perceived as rebelliousness but also found the laughter of the other children simply infuriating. As a punishment for her lack of conformity, the nun told Susan that she would have to spend a timeout in the supply closet.

At the end of the school day, Susan's mother was waiting outside the school, but her daughter did not come out. Much to the surprise of mother and teacher, poor Susan had been forgotten. She had spent hours in the closet, and her mother was understandably enraged. Adding to the pain of having been confined to the closet, Susan had urinated on herself and on the floor of the closet, and she felt utterly humiliated when the door was opened. Whereas Susan had previously enjoyed school, as a result of this experience, she developed an aversion to school, and there were daily struggles to get her to go. She then began to develop persistent problems of constipation, and in therapy, she reported painful memories of being held by her parents and having suppositories inserted on a regular basis.

I suggested EMDR to Susan to deal with the painful memories of the closet and suppositories. As is often seen in the efficient method of EMDR, Susan's painful memories and the perceptions of humiliation that accompanied them were transformed to the point at which she no longer felt unworthy, saw her teacher's actions as unintended, and stopped blaming her parents for what she had originally seen as a debasing and forced treatment of her constipation. Her progress in therapy was reflected in her taking better care of herself and presenting in a more self-assured manner. What did persist, however, were more general, free-floating anxiety and feelings of discomfort.

At this point, Susan agreed to try meditation to bring about a greater sense of tranquility and trust. The process started with a therapist-guided meditation, such as the mountain and lake meditations described earlier. This particular meditation was selected to counter her feelings of vulnerability and weakness, and replace them with perceptions of strength and endurance. Susan enjoyed meditation and took to it enthusiastically. Later approaches included the loving-kindness with a primary focus on self-acceptance and self-care. This movement from strength to self-acceptance, including acceptance of vulnerability, was especially helpful to her. Susan began using a phone application referred to as the "Calm app" and then began self-guided mindfulness practice, which she did regularly in the early morning and later in the day. She continued in therapy for approximately 6 months after beginning her meditations, and she did very well. Susan radiated contentment and confidence, and vowed to use her early painful experiences to help guide her in being an effective and caring teacher. Meditation appears to have become an integral part of life for Susan, and she has benefited from it exceedingly well. She has since left therapy, and occasional follow-ups reveal that she continues to do well.

WHAT IS THE EMPIRICAL SUPPORT FOR MEDITATION?

Empirical support exists for using meditation for treating PTSD and for reducing the anxiety and depression that accompany this disorder. The level of empirical support is not as strong as it is with EMDR and CBT-based interventions. The meta-analyses that have been conducted are supportive of this approach, but many of the studies lack the scientific rigor of randomized controlled trials, which may be partially due to the difficulty in designing such trials for this type of intervention. Given that the vast majority of U.S. Department of Veterans Affairs (VA) facilities support the use of meditation in treating trauma and that it has been shown to be effective with nonmilitary types of trauma should encourage treating clinicians to see meditation as a useful tool in trauma treatment.

In keeping with the theme of covering psychological interventions for PTSD for which there is empirical evidence, it does appear that the available research supports the utility of meditation. According to a meta-analysis by Hilton et al. (2017), three yoga, three MBSR, and two mantra repetition programs "reduced PTSD symptoms statistically significantly compared with all other comparators (TAU [treatment as usual] alone, education, or present-centered therapy) across all sources of trauma" (p. 459). A *mantra* is a sacred utterance—usually a word or group of words—often in Sanskrit believed to have psychological or spiritual powers, such as *Rama* (pronounced *RAH-mah*), which means eternal joy within and was Mahatma Gandhi's mantra (Hilton et al., 2017). So few studies were covered in this meta-analysis, however, because the analysis focused on randomized controlled studies of which there were few, and those that specifically focused on PTSD were even fewer. In another review (Kim, Schneider, Kravitz, Mermier, & Burge, 2013) 12 of 16 studies using mixed designs showed a positive effect of meditation on PTSD symptoms. Other reviews also showed promise for meditation compared with treatment as usual, attention matched controls, and active controls for treating PTSD (e.g., Vujanovic, Niles, Pietrefesa, Schmertz, & Potter, 2013).

According to Hilton et al. (2017), 89% of VA facilities use complementary and alternative therapeutic approaches, such as meditation. In a national sample of PTSD-diagnosed individuals, 39% reported use of these alternative methods (Libby, Pilver, & Desai, 2012). What these statistics suggest is that there is a demand for complementary and alternative medicine methods for treating PTSD. In addition, these methods show value in reducing the depression and anxiety that accompany PTSD, which is of no small significance because before the 2013 publication of the *Diagnostic and Statistical Manual of Mental Disorders* (fifth ed. [*DSM–5*]; American Psychiatric Association, 2013), PTSD was listed under the anxiety disorders in the fourth edition of the *DSM* (fourth ed. [*DSM–IV*]; American Psychiatric Association, 1994). Depression, anxiety, and PTSD are highly correlated with each other, so it is certainly possible that using complementary and alternative medicine procedures will reduce all three. The relatively high dropout rate from traditional exposure and CBT procedures (Schottenbauer, Glass, Arnkoff, Tendick, & Gray, 2008) provides a rationale for having alternative methods, and VA's heavy use of such methods should be evidence for their utility.

Another point to consider is that specific therapeutic approaches such as CBT and exposure therapy target symptoms, and again recall that symptom reduction is the basis of the medical model on which many psychological interventions are developed. But symptom reduction may be only half the battle. Many people with PTSD have a primary symptom of anxiety. If an intervention reduces anxiety, this does not mean that other deficient aspects of the sufferer's life will suddenly return to normal. Many of those suffering from PTSD have, in addition to anxiety, difficulties with social interaction, overuse of legal and illegal drugs, employment problems, concentration problems, and isolation. Meditations, such as loving-kindness, might be of value in allowing the PTSD sufferer to have more positive interactions with other people, which can have a snowball effect on addressing their other deficiencies. So, for example, mindfulness meditation increases the focus on the present and reduces obsessive worrying and rumination. By being present, one is less isolated and has the potential to be more socially engaged. Assuming a nonjudgmental stance like what takes place in meditation can help to reduce some of the suspiciousness that accompanies threats to oneself, and this reduction in negativistic thinking can also foster improved social interactions. Even with the potentially more general impact of mindfulness in comparison to CBT symptom-oriented interventions, the PTSD sufferer may still need employment counseling and assistance in reengaging in the world. Some (e.g., Hoge, 2011) have suggested that mindfulness be added to standard interventions such as CBT because mindfulness increases overall level of adaptability.

In a review of 12 studies (Banks, Newman, & Saleem, 2015), many of which lacked methodological rigor, the majority showed reductions in PTSD symptoms following mindfulness meditation interventions. These studies included a mix of randomized controlled trials, controlled trials, cohort studies, and observational studies. This review concluded that "mindfulness based interventions may be useful to decrease PTSD symptoms, in particular avoidance" (p. 959). This reduction in avoidance is an important finding. As I indicated earlier, avoidance is a major obstacle in treating PTSD. The anxiety that traditional interventions bring about is the major reason that traumatized individuals terminate treatment or don't seek it in the first place. If mindfulness can indeed have a positive impact in reducing avoidance, it will facilitate compliance and thereby reduce the suffering caused by PTSD.

One of the limitations cited in the Banks et al. (2015) review was the heterogeneous nature of the included samples. Some (e.g., Amstadter & Vernon, 2008) have suggested that exposure to different types of traumatic events, whether war, rape, car accident, or abuse, may result in varying posttraumatic reactions, including a speculated exacerbation of problems. However, despite the different types of trauma, these differences did not appear to influence the overall efficacy of the mindfulness intervention. Additional problematic issues were variations in the length of time since the trauma, the small sample sizes of some of the studies, and that several of the participants in the studies were in ongoing psychotherapy. Banks et al. suggested that future studies should have larger sample sizes, randomization with control groups, and, to more accurately gauge the impact of mindfulness, not have participants who are also engaged in therapy.

SUMMARY

A good deal of evidence shows that mindfulness meditation seems to be riding a wave, or perhaps a tsunami, of popularity. One sees the application of mindfulness interventions not just to trauma and PTSD but also to drug dependence, relationship and awareness enhancement, improvements in immune functioning, weight loss, and just about every other issue of concern to humanity. Empirical evidence shows that it beneficially impacts trauma. Earlier, I drew a distinction between efficacy and effectiveness. Efficacy is relevant to samples in controlled studies and effectiveness refers to usage within the noncircumscribed general population. When Western-trained clinicians and researchers evaluate the utility of interventions, they are usually examining the issue of efficacy. They want to know whether the intervention is "better than" a comparison intervention (e.g., treatment as usual). The way this is done, or is expected to be done, is to randomly assign participants to the intervention under investigation or to a control or comparison group of some kind, or both. In proceeding in this way, one then looks at outcome measures. These measures are expected to be psychometrically defensible (i.e., to be both reliable and valid).

But in proceeding this way, clinicians and researchers must ask ourselves: Are we attempting to squeeze an ill-defined experiential process through the eye of an experimental needle? Certainly, the aforementioned reviews provide evidence suggesting that mindfulness meditation has utility in improving specified symptoms, and that is an important finding. But it is not the only finding worth noting. Various writers have spoken about self-transformations, increased levels of compassion, and an evolving nonjudgmental stance, all of which occur through meditative practice and are not so readily measurable through the use of tight experimental designs.

Langer (2014) provided a humorous, although telling, fable that suggests that we might be "missing the forest for the trees" as far as mindfulness is concerned: Three researchers took up residence on a very small atoll to study pure animal behavior. They had been there many years, were completely cut off from society, and resembled hermits. One day, a learned psychometrician stopped by the island to help these hermit-researchers recall some of the statistical methods they had forgotten and that would be needed should they wish to publish their findings in a refereed scientific journal. Langer continued the story:

> So, the wise doctor spoke to them for many hours, reviving their memories of simple and complex designs, of methods and techniques necessary for publication and instructed them so they could recognize the proper statistical test for their data once more. (p. 201)

While getting ready to leave the island by boat, the doctor of statistics saw something surprising. A rhesus monkey was riding on the back of a large porpoise that was approaching his craft. On pulling alongside, the monkey called out:

Dear and wise Professor, we have been trained in the laboratory . . . and they [the researchers] crave your forgiveness for sending us to trouble you with their difficulty, but none of them can remember how you said to determine the denominator degrees of freedom, and since they must know this in order to get their results published. (Langer, 2014, p. 202)

It appears the researchers had not noticed the monkeys could talk, and so it may be with mindfulness. We may be focused on the mundane and ignoring the momentous. We emphasize and focus on the reduction of PTSD symptoms while not seeing that meditation can create an openness of awareness and a greater sense of compassion and caring for self and others.

5

Exercise, Trauma, and Negative Emotional States

Considerable literature shows that exercise can lower anxiety, depression, and other negative emotions. This chapter addresses the newly discovered impact of exercise on PTSD. Exercise has been found to reduce PTSD in children, adolescents, and adults.

EFFECT OF EXERCISE ON ADULT PTSD

If you had asked me back in 2000 whether exercise could be of any value for the treatment of posttraumatic stress disorder (PTSD), my answer would clearly have been no. At that time, I believed that exercise, particularly aerobic exercise, was helpful in moderating emotional states such as anxiety and depression because I had been involved in a series of early studies to support this stance (e.g., Altchiler & Motta, 1994; Stein & Motta, 1992). However, there was virtually no evidence of its utility in managing PTSD. My reasoning was that PTSD is a far more complex disorder than many of the emotional disorders. It transforms the individual sufferer on nearly all levels. It is not as simple as fear of driving on highways but involves an alteration of one's sense

Portions of this chapter have been adapted from "The Role of Exercise in Reducing PTSD and Negative Emotional States" [Open access peer-reviewed chapter], by R. Motta in *Psychology of Health—Biopsychosocial Approach*, by S. G. Taukeni (Ed.), 2018, London, United Kingdom: IntechOpen. Copyright 2018 by R. Motta. Retrieved from https://www.intechopen.com/books/psychology-of-health-biopsychosocial-approach/the-role-of-exercise-in-reducing-ptsd-and-negative-emotional-states.

http://dx.doi.org/10.1037/0000186-006
Alternative Therapies for PTSD: The Science of Mind–Body Treatments, by R. W. Motta

of self and one's view of the environment. At the Child and Family Trauma Institute that I direct and in my clinical practice, PTSD sufferers report that they are no longer the person they once were and they no longer see the world in the same way. This is exactly what I told Theresa Manger when she asked me to mentor her on her doctoral dissertation involving the impact of exercise on PTSD, anxiety, and depression. As it turned out, I was wrong. Her successful dissertation defense and subsequent publication proved that her instincts were correct (Manger & Motta, 2005). To say that I was surprised by her results is the very definition of understatement.

In her study, Manger (Manger & Motta, 2005) obtained a sample of individuals from the community through advertisements and fliers seeking those willing to participate in a study investigating the relationship between trauma-related stress and exercise. We expected that participants had not engaged in regular physical exercise for 1 month before the study, they were not on any form of psychotropic medication, they had written medical approval from a physician to engage in an exercise program, they were willing to participate in a 10-week exercise study, they were not a substance abuser, and they did not exhibit psychosis or gross psychopathology, such as schizophrenia. The traumatic events of the final sample who participated in the study included tragic death of a loved one or friend, sexual or physical assault, serious accident (most common were automobile accidents), combat, severe illness or disease, or injury. Study participants who were, on average, 48 years of age, reported experiencing between two and six traumatic events. We built in a 1-month follow-up period after the exercise intervention to rule out the possibility that factors such as social interaction during exercise, eagerness to please the researchers, or novelty effects may have been responsible for any results we obtained.

To see what changes occur over time in individuals who have mild or higher levels of PTSD, we assigned participants to a 5- or 10-week baseline period in which they did not engage in exercise but were simply monitored on standardized measures of PTSD, anxiety, and depression (Manger & Motta, 2005). Following the end of the baseline periods, study participants began a manualized exercise program administered at a local YMCA. The manual required a warm-up of 5 minutes of bicycling and 5 minutes of stretching. Participants were then required to walk or jog on a treadmill at a moderate intensity level for 30 minutes followed by a cooldown period of 10 minutes, and then required to stretch and bicycle again. *Moderate-intensity exercise* was defined as 60% to 80% of maximum heart rate for half an hour (Bushman, 2017). Heart rate monitors were provided. Participants agreed to exercise two to three times per week for 10 weeks. The minimum was 12 exercise sessions over 10 weeks. We administered assessment measures at the beginning of baseline, end of baseline, end of exercise intervention, and follow-up.

Overall, results showed significant reductions in PTSD, anxiety, and depression following the exercise intervention (Manger & Motta, 2005). These results were maintained during the 1-month follow-up period. We came to realize that community interventions such as this exercise program could be an important resource for trauma victims who do not traditionally seek help. Help-seeking often involves the perceived stigma of being involved in psychotherapy, aversion to the use of psychotropic medications, concern about medication side effects, and fear of incurring burdensome costs. In addition, the tendency to avoid directly dealing with one's traumatic experiences at all costs is ever present.

In the exercise intervention (Manger & Motta, 2005) presented, participants did not need to deal with traumatic experiences other than what they may have been encountered when filling out paper-and-pencil measures of trauma and answering questions during initial interview. We cannot attribute the reductions in negative emotional states that followed the exercise intervention to any traditional form of therapeutic intervention because none was offered in this study. It appeared that exercise alone was responsible for the reductions in PTSD, anxiety, and depression. This finding, of course, begs the question, which may be unanswerable: Why does exercise have a beneficial effect as just noted? To date, there seems to be no universally agreed on answer. Nevertheless, abundant empirical support now exists for using exercise as an intervention for PTSD. In the following sections, I review the relevant studies in some detail owing to the importance of using exercise as both a therapeutic adjunct and, in many cases, as a standalone intervention for PTSD. Reviews are also available (e.g., Motta, 2018a, 2018b).

WHY DOES EXERCISE HELP WITH PTSD AND EMOTIONAL DISORDERS?

The short answer to this question is that no one knows for sure why exercise is beneficial in reducing PTSD and the anxiety and depression that accompany this disorder. A number of hypotheses have been put forth, such as thermogenic hypothesis, endorphin and endocannabinoid hypotheses, monoamine hypothesis, distraction hypothesis, and self-efficacy theory. All have adherents, but no one hypothesis has been universally accepted.

Thermogenic Hypothesis

Thermogenic hypothesis proposes that exercise creates an elevation in body temperature, resulting in a beneficial impact on emotional states (e.g., DeBoer, Powers, Utschig, Otto, & Smits, 2012). Specifically, aerobic forms of exercise are said to raise the temperature of brain regions, such as the brain stem, thus producing a tranquilizing effect along with muscle tension reduction. Adherents to the hypothesis have used it specifically to explain anxiety reduction rather than reduction of depression and PTSD symptoms (Motta, 2018b). However, given that PTSD was formerly classified as an anxiety disorder, and anxiety is a major component of PTSD, it stands to reason that exercise would have a beneficial impact on PTSD.

One of the difficulties with the thermogenic hypothesis is that temperature elevation might be an intervening variable that has little to do with the beneficial emotional impact of exercise. For example, it may be that exercise increases temperature but also alters neurochemistry, and it is the change in neurochemistry that produces the benefit, not temperature elevation per se. From this perspective, temperature plays a correlational rather than a causal role. In addition, living in a warm environment has not been shown to reduce depression, anxiety, or PTSD, nor does having a fever, which also increases internal body temperature. The thermogenic hypothesis does not appear to have held up well as an explanation for the beneficial effects on emotion resulting from exercise.

Endorphin and Endocannabinoid Hypotheses

Perhaps the most popular explanation for the positive impact on mood that results from exercise is the *endorphin hypothesis* (e.g., Farrell, Gates, Maksud, & Morgan, 1982). This hypothesis is based on the observation that following vigorous exercise of a half hour or more, an elevation of a special endogenous opiate (β-, or beta-, endorphin) occurs. This endogenous or body-produced opiate is released through exercise, and some say it is responsible for the *runner's high*, an elevation of mood following running or jogging for extended periods (Motta, 2018b). The endorphin hypothesis is not without its critics who have carefully examined the data from empirical studies.

One such study (Alfermann & Stoll, 2005) compared a jogging group with a relaxation group that did not engage in exercise and with a group that did back stretches. The moods examined were anger, tension, energy level, calmness, positive mood, depression, and others. Although all groups produced positive emotional changes, the researchers found no differences among the groups. If beta-endorphin is released through exercise, the nonexercise groups should not have shown positive changes, and yet they did. Clearly something other than, or in addition to, endorphins must be responsible for positive emotional effects of exercise.

A further critique of the endorphin hypothesis is that circulating endorphin levels do not reflect brain endorphin levels, and endorphins cannot cross the blood–brain barrier. So, even if exercise increases circulating or peripheral endorphin levels, those increased levels should not have an impact on brain-mediated emotional states. Another criticism of the endorphin hypothesis is that when the endorphin-blocking substance naloxone, an opiate antagonist, is provided to those experiencing the runner's high, it does not diminish the elevation in mood. If endorphins were causal to exercise-induced mood changes, one would expect a significant deterioration in mood following naloxone injection (Motta, 2018b).

It may be of some significance to note that a recent alternative to the endorphin hypothesis has come to be known as the *endocannabinoid hypothesis* (Smaga, Bystrowska, Gawlinski, Przegalinski, & Filip, 2014). Endocannabinoids are substances produced by the body that are similar in action to that of tetrahydrocannabinol (THC), the active constituent in marijuana. Using trained male college students running on a treadmill or cycling on a stationary bike for 50 minutes at 70% to 80% of maximum heart rate, elevations of endocannabinoids were detected in blood plasma (Dietrich & McDaniel, 2004). Because activation of the endocannabinoid system reduces pain sensations, it has been suggested that it might be what is behind the runner's high and alterations of mental and emotional processes (Dietrich & McDaniel, 2004). Owing to the presence of cannabinoid receptors in the skin, lungs, and muscles, it is speculated that endocannabinoids may have a role in producing analgesic effects that occur through exercise. Unlike the endorphin hypothesis—recall that endorphins do not cross the blood–brain barrier—cannabinoids do appear to operate both centrally (i.e., in the central nervous system) and in the peripheral nervous system. They reportedly reduce anxiety, alter attention, and impair working memory much like THC does. So, although research is in the early phases, endocannabinoids have been proposed as an alternative to endorphins as the possible mediator of the runner's high, analgesic effects, and beneficial psychological effects of exercise. The endocannabinoid hypothesis was developed comparatively recently and is not anywhere near as widely accepted as the apparently doubtful endorphin hypothesis (Motta, 2018b).

Monoamine Hypothesis

The *monamine hypothesis* is somewhat like the endorphin and endocannabinoid hypotheses in that is proposes that exercise produces chemical changes in the body, and it is these alterations that cause mood changes in exercise (e.g., Lin & Kuo, 2013). The monoamine hypothesis proposes that exercise results in increased brain availability of brain neurotransmitters, such as serotonin, dopamine, and norepinephrine, and these neurotransmitters result in reductions in depression and other negative emotional states. Available studies (e.g., Lin & Kuo, 2013) show that although exercise does result in monoamine elevations as assessed in plasma and urine, the question remains whether similar elevations in the brain take place. Testing of biochemical hypotheses is difficult in humans because it often involves invasive procedures, such as spinal taps for cerebrospinal fluid samples. Furthermore, biochemical samples obtained from blood or other body fluids may not necessarily reflect the availability of similar biochemical samples in the brain. Animal studies suggest that exercise increases serotonin and norepinephrine in the brain, but reliable and replicable studies in humans have not demonstrated this finding with consistency (e.g., Patki et al., 2014).

Another line of reasoning that further clouds the issue of whether biochemical changes following exercise are causal of positive mood enhancement is that all mental activity is, in essence, chemical activity of the nervous system, especially the central nervous system (Motta, 2018b). So, as I soon discuss, it may be possible that positive mood states arise from perceptions of having successfully completed some form of strenuous activity, and the positive mental state is what drives the biochemical changes rather than the other way around. The issue is, What is responsible for causing what? Which came first?

Distraction Hypothesis

In accord with the preceding statements, the *distraction hypothesis* suggests that psychological or environmental changes are responsible for changes in emotional states following exercise and that biochemical mediators play an ancillary role (e.g., Peluso & Guerra de Andrade, 2005). The hypothesis proposes that when one is engaged in vigorous physical activity, it is difficult to simultaneously entertain depressive thoughts and negatively tinged ruminations and preoccupations. People only have so much attention to go around, and when one is busy exercising, little attention is available for depressive rumination. Usually when one is inactive and immobile, and has few demands on one's time, time and space are available to engage in depressive thoughts. And, as discussed earlier, negative thinking and cognitive distortions are the basis for negative emotional states, according to cognitive behavior therapy (CBT) perspectives.

In some studies (e.g., Alfermann & Stoll, 2005), exercise has been compared with control groups, such as relaxation, training, or wait-list controls, in which one is distracted yet not involved in physical activity. The results of these studies are varied: Some show reductions in depression following distracting activity, and some do not. However, when one examines mood elevation and not simply reduction in depression, usually exercise shows greater changes than nonexercise interventions. So, it is possible that distraction serves as a means through which one moves away from depressive rumination, but that for mood elevation to occur, distraction may not be a sufficient means in and of itself.

Self-Efficacy Theory

Self-efficacy perceptions refer to one's self-view of their capabilities to accomplish certain objectives. The originator of *self-efficacy theory* (Bandura, 1997) claimed that people who are depressed are comparatively lacking in a healthy sense of self-efficacy. Those who are clinically depressed see themselves as relatively incapable of setting goals and accomplishing hoped for objectives. These negative self-perceptions eventuate in depressive rumination on, for example, perceived inadequacies, and these perceptions decrease the possibility of engaging in self-validating behaviors.

The studies that have been conducted (e.g., Bodin & Martinsen, 2004) do show that when one engages in physical exercise, they feel more accomplished and more capable of achieving various exercise-related goals. Their self-efficacy perceptions (i.e., their view of themselves setting specific exercise targets and accomplishing them) has been found to increase following a planned sequence of exercise. The research, however, on whether these enhanced views of exercise competence can produce reductions in clinical depression is less clear-cut. What does seem clear is that exercise is associated with reductions in depression and elevation in mood. Whether these outcomes result from alterations in one's self-perceptions of their capabilities is less obvious (Motta, 2018b).

Conclusion Regarding Causal Hypotheses of Exercise Effects

It is unclear whether biochemical or psychological factors mediate the positive effects of exercise on mood states, such as depression. Depression and anxiety are significant factors in PTSD, and the alleviation of the emotional distress they cause would be a productive step in treating PTSD. Perhaps clinicians and researchers are making an error in seeking out unitary causes for the beneficial effects of exercise and that a combination of biochemistry, psychology, and maybe even socialization, and, in some instances, even spiritual issues, come into play. Maybe these causes vary in importance depending on at what point in one's cycle of emotional distress one chooses to intervene (Motta, 2018b). What one can derive from the available literature is that exercise alleviates emotional distress and has been found to play a significant role in reducing PTSD. Why this is so is, as of this writing, unclear.

FROM RESEARCH TO CLINICAL PERSPECTIVES

Those clinicians who have treated individuals suffering from PTSD, anxiety, and depression know that it is challenging to get them to engage in exercise despite its beneficial effects. Bushman (2017) recommends that individuals between the ages of 18 and 65 should engage in moderate-intensity exercise for 30 minutes, 5 days a week (Motta, 2018b). As mentioned earlier in the chapter, moderate-intensity exercise is 60% to 80% of maximum heart rate (Bushman, 2017). In general, maximum heart rate has been calculated as 220 minus age multiplied by .6 to .8. So, for an individual who is 50, the calculation would be $220 - 50 = 170$; $170 \times (.6) = 102$; $170 \times (.8) = 136$ (Motta, 2018b). Therefore, the 50-year-old should exercise in such a way that they maintain a heart rate of 102 to 136 for half an hour, 5 days a week. Is this reasonable?

These numbers—exercising 5 days a week for 30 minutes at moderate intensity—are, for all intents and purposes, unrealistic for many and especially for people who are depressed. Getting a depressed client to do anything, other than what is absolutely necessary to get on with their lives, is often a real challenge. So, what is realistic? Frequently, just getting them to go for a walk for 10 minutes or so maybe twice a week might be a major accomplishment. Because most emotionally troubled clients are not physically fit, are unmotivated, and are resistant to physical activity, the idea is to start at a nonchallenging level (Motta, 2018b). Be encouraging and increase of level of exercise slowly. The guiding principle is the following: Take baby steps. Start emotionally distressed clients with something they might view as enjoyable. A 10-minute stroll in the park might be a suitable starting point. Certainly, a moderate-to-vigorous intensity level three to five times per week is likely to have a psychologically beneficial effect, but if the exercise demands become overwhelming to a client, which they easily can, not only will the client become discouraged, but they may also begin to believe that their therapist does not understand them and is out of touch. The client may see their inability to accomplish exercise goals as a failure, and this failure further validates a negative, depressive self-view. As in treating PTSD, the mantra is as follows: Move slowly and at a pace the client can tolerate.

CASE EXAMPLE: ADVISING A DEPRESSED CLIENT TO ENGAGE IN EXERCISE

As many clinicians will assert, it is often difficult to determine whether exercise had a beneficial impact because it frequently is combined with other interventions. This case involving Mary, who was diagnosed with PTSD, is a somewhat typical example of the complexities of prescribing exercise as an intervention for depression but also highlights the difficulty in evaluating the effectiveness of this intervention. Often a client such as Mary is engaging in psychotherapy in which the focus is on elevating her sense of self-esteem, improving her perceptions of self-efficacy, and basically providing validation for the choices she has made. All the while, the client is being prescribed different psychotropic medications and acceding to the therapist's requests to stay active, be socially engaged, and exercise. So, determining which of these interventions or which combinations of interventions leads to desirable outcomes is difficult, to say the least. Often, the only data the clinician has are the client's self-reports of what they saw as beneficial.

At the time I saw her, Mary was a 53-year-old mother of two children, both of whom had recently completed college. She and her husband were employed by a large utility company; he, in a supervisory capacity. Mary had worked at this company for nearly 30 years, enjoyed her work, and felt that she was effective and well regarded. She reported never having been a depressive type and to have been physically and socially active. Unexpectedly, her company offered what seemed to be a generous early retirement package. It appeared that the company was becoming far more computer oriented and expected employees to either become adept at new computerized systems or go for early retirement and allow other, younger, tech-savvy individuals to take their place. Mary decided to not take what was offered in the hope that the company would present an even more generous incentive package. She believed she might be able to acquire the necessary computer skills in the unlikely event that a more generous retirement incentive did not become available. However, no further incentive package was offered, and the company had withdrawn the initial one for anyone who had not taken it. Acquiring the needed computer skills turned out to be more of a challenge than Mary expected.

She reported that this situation was traumatizing to her, and she did show classic PTSD symptoms of sleeplessness, withdrawal from others, preoccupation with not being valued at work, and a generally negative view of herself and her future. She also began to view herself as having made a terrible decision, and over a succession of weeks, Mary started to redevelop neck pain from an old auto accident injury and to become increasingly depressed. She saw a doctor who put her on pain medication, prescribed steroid injections, and recommended bed rest. Her company agreed that work would be too stressful for her and allowed her a temporary medical leave. While at home, Mary began ruminating about her decision to "not take the package" and would spend endless hours essentially beating herself up psychologically for having made an "idiotic decision." Her sense of self-worth sank to unfamiliar low levels, and she spent most of her days in bed, in her pajamas, either watching TV or sleeping. She began to look haggard and, after a while, rarely came out of her bedroom. At the recommendation of her general practitioner, she began to take Ambien (zolpidem tartrate) for sleep difficulties and Xanax (alprazolam) for anxiety. Her doctor subsequently added Lexapro (escitalopram oxalate), an antidepressant.

When I saw Mary for the first time—in the waiting room—she looked lifeless. She had dark circles under her eyes, spoke in a barely audible tone, and generally came across as emotionally flat and exhausted. She was a frightening sight. She seemed an empty shell.

In our first session, I strongly recommended that she get back to exercising. She used to routinely jog and now did nothing to stay fit. I reviewed and summarized empirical studies showing that exercise could have a remarkably beneficial effect on negative moods and could actually enhance positive mood states. At first, Mary took my suggestions to exercise with a "yes-but" stance: "Yes, but my neck is hurting. I don't have a gym membership. The weather is too cold. I don't have the energy. I don't have the time." And yet she had plenty of time to ruminate. I pointed out that she used to be a regular jogger to encourage her to begin to exercise for brief periods using a treadmill.

Mary complied and started a treadmill routine of at least a half hour per day at varying levels of intensity. Over a period of several months, Mary began showing significant reductions in depression, which, as I indicated earlier, is a critical component in PTSD. She also started looking younger, became more upbeat, and seemed a more vibrant person. By her own account, she is still not completely out of the woods because she occasionally finds herself ruminating and beating herself up. However, overall, she has made wonderful progress, is more hopeful, and continues to be committed to regular exercise.

And now we get to the point of trying to figure out what led to her improvement. So many factors were involved:

- I challenged Mary's self-downing cognitions, and she and I practiced more objective ways of interpreting what had taken place at work.

- Mary came to believe that her decision to hold out for a better deal was a quite normal response.

- She began an exercise program that she was initially reluctant to initiate but subsequently embraced with gusto.

- Mary started going to church almost daily and took comfort in sermons and prayers.

- Mary's husband proved to be supportive: He states he will stand by her regardless of whether she chooses to go back to work or simply quits and takes early retirement.

- Mary has been socializing more with friends.

- She has made every effort to stay active and catch herself when she sees depressive rumination reoccur.

- Mary is continuing to take a low dosage of antidepressant medication.

So, was it a combination of all of these factors that led her out of the depths of depression and PTSD? When I asked Mary what, in her view, led to change, she targeted exercise and church attendance. Perhaps she is right, and we really have no way of knowing, but exercise was clearly was an important part of her recovery.

The reader may recall a study presented earlier (Motta & Lynch, 1990) in which youths showed significant improvement in behavior following a behaviorally oriented approach to therapy. Parents saw the relationship with the therapist as precipitating positive changes. Therapists saw therapeutic techniques as the reason for positive outcomes. Sometimes it is impossible to know for sure what actually was responsible for positive change in cases such as Mary's. Nevertheless, what is known through numerous empirical studies is that exercise has a positive impact in reducing depression and other disorders, such as anxiety and PTSD. Regardless of the nature of the causal chain, I highly recommend making physical activity an adjunctive or central part of most therapeutic endeavors when negative emotional states are the areas of concern. Abundant research shows the beneficial impact of exercise on negative emotional states, and I review some of this research in detail, as follows, because of its importance to clinical practice.

RESEARCH SUPPORTING EXERCISE AS A PTSD TREATMENT

The recognition that exercise can be a useful tool in reducing PTSD symptoms is a fairly recent development. Abundant research validates the usefulness of exercise in reducing negative emotional states like anxiety and depression.

It is possible that because anxiety and depression play such a key role in PTSD that their reduction may explain the improvements in PTSD symptoms following exercise.

Empirical Studies of Exercise and PTSD

Shivakumar, Anderson, Surís, and North (2017) conducted a study of adults in which they focused specifically on women veterans of childbearing age to determine if exercise alone could positively affect PTSD. The exercise intervention took place at a facility housed in the Veterans Affairs Medical Center in Dallas, Texas. As part of the exercise protocol, participants walked at a rate of 3 miles per hour—at a brisk pace along a grade—for 30 to 40 minutes, 4 days a week, for a total of 12 weeks. Gradually, during the first 3 weeks, the duration of exercise increased so that it was at full duration of 30 to 40 minutes per session by the end of Week 3. Exercise sessions involved a 3- to 5-minute warm-up before study participants then increased their walking speed to the targeted level of intensity. About 75% of participants finished the 12-week exercise program. These completion and attrition rates are comparable with using yoga as an intervention for women with PTSD, meaning that both yoga and exercise are readily tolerated.

Results showed significant reductions in PTSD and depression, as well as increases in quality of life measures and pain reduction. Concluded Shivakumar et al. (2017): "Finally, for patients with prominent avoidance related to their traumatic events, exercise many provide a safe and structured activity than can address social isolation and promote recovery" (p. 1813). As I mention earlier in this book, avoidance is a major problem in treating PTSD. If such interventions as exercise, meditation, and yoga can be effective in reducing this disorder and do not heavily emphasize having to repeatedly confronting prior trauma, they have an important place in clinicians' treatment choices (Motta, 2018b). No study, though, is without limitations, including this one by Shivakumar et al., which did not include a comparison group that was diagnosed with PTSD but was not receiving exercise. Notwithstanding, the overall thrust of existing empirical studies seems to point to exercise as an effective intervention for PTSD.

The majority of research studies on exercise and PTSD, including those I have presented so far, used a cross-sectional approach: A group of individuals—typically adults—with PTSD are enrolled in an exercise program for a specific period; the researcher(s) given the participants pre- and posttest measures to determine if reductions in negative emotional states have occurred. In contrast Whitworth, Craft, Dunsiger, and Ciccolo (2017) conducted an online longitudinal study involving 182 individuals who screened positive for PTSD. Participant completed not only a measure of PTSD but also online assessments of exercise behavior, psychological distress, sleep quality, pain, and alcohol or substance abuse. The authors found a significant and direct effect of total leisure-time exercise on avoidance or *numbing*—emotional dampening and lack of engagement—symptoms of PTSD. This finding was of no small significance because avoidance is the major stumbling block in treating people who are traumatized (Motta, 2018b). For those engaged in *strenuous intensity exercise*, which the study defined as vigorous running or cycling, the authors (Whitworth et al., 2017) found significantly less avoidance or numbing and hyperarousal. Compared to study participants who were less active, those who engaged in strenuous exercise activity also reported a reduction in overall PTSD symptoms, better sleep quality, a decrease in pain, and reduced substance abuse (Motta, 2018b).

After the study ended, the authors (Whitworth et al., 2017) speculated that sufficiently intense exercise of adequate duration might lead to one's becoming accustomed to the physical stressors of exercise. Subsequently, in response to stressors such as those associated with PTSD, this habituation might result in an adaptation in stress response and fewer negative cognitive appraisals (Whitworth et al., 2017). The reexperiencing of stressors is common among PTSD sufferers. If the stress response can be dampened as it appears to be when exercising vigorously, it is possible to have a spillover effect into the cognitive domain, whereby memories of trauma may then evoke fewer of the negative cognitions seen in PTSD.

Overall results of the Whitworth et al. (2017) study point to beneficial effects of aerobic activity, particularly for those who exercise vigorously. However, one should not interpret this conclusion to mean that moderate levels of exercise are not of value. The general message from the research literature is that even moderate levels of exercise are effective in reducing both anxiety and depression (Motta, 2018b). Given that anxiety and depression are key components of PTSD, it should be clear that encouraging clients to exercise is excellent practice.

Some (e.g., Cirrik & Hacioglu, 2016) claim that the beneficial effects of exercise may result from changes in brain morphology, chemistry, and function. These beneficial effects include improved learning and memory, antidepressant and antianxiety effects, reduced cognitive decline related to aging, and improvements in symptoms of neurodegenerative diseases. Exercise appears to improve mood and cognition, and it has its greatest effects on the hippocampus, where both neurogenesis (nerve cell growth) and angiogenesis (increase blood availability through the growth of new blood vessels) have been shown. Although further research is needed into the exact molecular mechanisms responsible for the exercise-induced neuroplasticity, progress is continuing in this area, especially regarding studies of neurotransmitter systems (Motta, 2018b).

A study by de Moor, Beem, Stubbe, Boomsma, and De Geus (2006) examined active and inactive young adult twins with diagnosable anxiety disorders and PTSD. They found that exercise reduced anxiety, PTSD, agoraphobia, and other specific phobias in the physically active twin. Twins who did not engage in exercise did not have reductions in these disorders. The value of this study is that it helps nullify genetic explanations of why individuals may benefit from exercise. The authors kept the genetic factor relatively constant and continued to find that exercise alone benefited the active twin.

Exercise and PTSD in Adolescents

All of the aforementioned studies involved investigations of the psychological effects of exercise with adults. The next step was to determine if the same positive outcomes of exercise would occur in an adolescent sample. A colleague and I (Newman & Motta, 2007) recruited participants from a residential treatment center: They were female; had primarily been physically abused, sexually abused, or maltreated, or some combination of those; were between the ages of 14 and 17; and had a diagnosis of PTSD based on standardized measures. Participants engaged in a structured group aerobic exercise program for 40 minutes, three times per week, for a total of 8 weeks. The form of exercise varied: Some girls jogged and others did kickboxing, but both forms produced an aerobic effect. We took measures of PTSD, anxiety, and depression twice during the beginning and end of a baseline period in which no intervention occurred, at the end of the exercise intervention, and at a 1-month follow-up. Once again, results provided support for the positive effects of aerobic exercise on reducing PTSD, anxiety, and depression. Fewer of the youth participants met the criteria for PTSD at the end of the study than at the beginning, and overall, the study showed significant reductions in anxiety and depression.

One of the major values of the exercise intervention is that it achieved positive therapeutic outcomes without the need for the adolescents to engage in formal therapy, which they were reluctant to do (Motta, 2018b). The adolescent females may have been immensely troubled by their abuse and thus may have avoided sharing information in a formal therapeutic setting. If significant symptom reduction can be attained by a simple aerobic exercise activity, such activity should become part of the formal structure of interventions for these youths.

Finding that simple aerobic exercise interventions could reduce PTSD within adult and adolescent samples, another colleague and I (Diaz & Motta, 2008) conducted a study with youths ages 14 to 17 years of age who lived in a private residential treatment facility. This time, though, the authors attempted to use only moderate-intensity walking as the form of intervention rather than forms of more intense aerobic activity as was done in the prior research project (Newman & Motta, 2007). In this (Diaz & Motta, 2008) study, participants completed a 5-week baseline and then an intervention involving 25-minute sessions of exercise that included 1 minute of slow leisurely walking (warm-up), 23 minutes of moderate-intensity walking, and 1 minute of slow leisurely walking (cooldown). Heart rates were maintained at 60% to 90% of maximum. By keeping the intervention unvaried and structured, the hope was to make the study more precise than earlier conducted investigations. The majority of participants showed statistically significant reductions in PTSD symptoms from baseline to postintervention. We (Diaz & Motta, 2008) also found a reduction in trauma-related stress. Results of anxiety and depression measures were not as clear-cut as those from PTSD perhaps because initial levels were not overly high, thus significant reductions were less likely to occur (Motta, 2018b). Like previous studies, the reductions in PTSD were primarily maintained in follow-up, and in some cases, the reductions became more pronounced over time.

We (Diaz & Motta, 2008) concluded that aerobic exercise interventions might be appropriate for youths who demonstrate difficulty expressing their emotions verbally as is required in traditional CBT-type therapies. In addition, aerobic exercise as an intervention for PTSD may be more appropriate than exposure therapies in that it is more likely to be tolerated in teens who have difficulty maintaining self-control, concentration problems, and histories of sexual abuse and avoidance of discussing their traumatic experiences that such abuse usually produces.

In another study involving adolescent females, Silvestri (2001) suggested that peer pressures related to social acceptance significantly affects the high level of anxiety in this group. Peers judged the merit of these participants based on such factors as wearing fashionable clothes, having a boyfriend, doing well in school, and being popular. In the study, individuals in the exercise group participated in 50-minute dance classes, four times a week for 4 weeks. The classes followed a dance routine to elevate heart rate to 160 beats per minute and ended with a cooldown to bring the heart rate down to 100 beats per minute. Results showed clear benefits of engaging in the aerobic dance routine to reduce anxiety. Thus, it appears that a variety of exercises from treadmills, to walking, to kickboxing, to dance, and others can have beneficial effects on negative emotional states.

CHILDHOOD ANXIETY AND PTSD REDUCTION THROUGH EXERCISE

With the exception of the few studies just described that involve older children and early adolescents, not many studies have examined the impact of exercise, anxiety, depression, and PTSD in children, and yet anxiety and depression are key components of PTSD (Motta, 2018b). In commenting on the effects of exercise on anxiety, Paluska and Schwenk (2000) noted that only about 36% of children and adolescents participate in physical education, which is unfortunate given the beneficial effects that exercise appears to have in relation to emotional disorders. An exercise—anxiety reduction relationship is evident in the few exercise interventions that have been implemented with children; Berk (2007) attributed these positive changes to endorphin release through exercise and also found a correlation between exercise and improved social skills, decreased negative thoughts, and boosts in self-confidence, as have I (Motta, McWilliams, Schwartz, & Cavera, 2012).

Although correlational relationships exist between anxiety reduction and exercise, one question is whether the measures used are appropriate for children because most have been normed on adult samples. Because children and adolescents do not accurately report the levels at which they exercise, research involving these populations is challenging (Motta et al., 2012). Parfitt and Eston (2005) stated that children and adolescents ages 11 to 13 years remembered less than half of the activities they engaged in during each day of school. These authors suggested using objective measures, including measurements of body fat, heart rate monitors, and pedometers. They also suggested that when such reliable measurements are used, the relationship between exercise and anxiety reduction shows itself to be as valid in children and adolescents as in adults.

In a study involving children, Annesi (2005) conducted a controlled investigation in which 9- to 12-year-olds engaged in 12 weeks of physical activity, resistance training, and stretching. Exercise resulted in reduced anxiety and negative mood, and improvements in physical and overall self-concept. Additional studies have correlated exercise among children with improvements in grades, standardized test scores, and feelings of well-being (Motta, 2018b).

Overall, the comparatively few studies conducted with children have consistently revealed a pattern of statistically significant relationships between exercise and reduction in anxiety (Motta et al., 2012). Although one can critique virtually all individual studies on methodological grounds, including sampling problems, lack of random assignment, and psychometric weakness of the measures used, the overall thrust of the published research is that exercise, particularly aerobic exercise, lowers anxiety levels. The existence of physical fitness programs within schools appears to result in muscle and cardiopulmonary improvements, and also to have a beneficial impact on mood states. Budgetary constraints often have a negative impact on such programs. Given the available research on the benefits of exercise, it would behoove school boards to give higher priority to physical fitness programs within the public and private school systems.

Exercise and Depression in Child and Adolescent Samples

Hundreds of empirical studies have found that exercise significantly reduces depression in adult samples, frequently to a degree equal to or greater than traditional cognitive therapies (e.g., Mulcahy, 1998) and psychotropic medication (Motta, 2018b). Undoubtedly, exercise is a useful adjunct to traditional therapies or as a stand-alone intervention for reducing depression. The problem, though, with prescribing exercise—as clinicians are all too well aware—is that the more depressed a person is, the less likely they are to engage in exercise. They simply lack energy or motivation to travel to a gym or go outside and engage in brisk walking, jogging, or swimming. The research on childhood and adolescent depression is far less abundant than that of adults (Motta, 2018b).

Children and adolescents who are depressed experience prolonged or temporary sadness, reduced interest in normal activity, negative and self-critical self-evaluation, difficulties in concentration and memory, socialization difficulties, and impairment in everyday functioning. In the United States, up to 2.5% of children and 8.3% of adolescents suffer from depression (Motta, 2018b). The problems of depressed youths can extend well past childhood and lead to substance abuse and suicide. Approximately 7% of adolescents who develop major depressive disorder later commit suicide as young adults (National Institute of Mental Health, 2000). Research suggests that in addition to the treatment options of traditional psychotherapies and medication, physical activity is an alternative for these youths.

In a correlational study, Field, Diego, and Sanders (2001) examined the relationships among self-reported exercise levels; depression; and a number of other interpersonal characteristics, such as relationships with parents and peers, sports involvement, drug use, and academic performance. A sample of high school seniors completed questionnaires and, on the basis of their answers, the authors divided them into two groups: low exercise and high exercise. Findings showed that the high-exercise group reported significantly less depression, lower drug use, and better relationships than the low-exercise group. Although exercise appeared to produce these positive outcomes, one could argue that those who were less depressed were more likely to have already been engaging in these positive behaviors, unlike the previously depressed individuals (Motta, 2018b). The problems establishing causality from correlational studies are well known.

In contrast to the Field et al. (2001) correlational study, typical experimental studies randomly assign participants into groups: those who receive treatment and those who do not. The researchers gather data before and after the intervention, and compare the participants' results to one another. Doing so allows them to make inferences about the effects of the treatment, in this case, exercise, on depressive symptomology (Motta, 2018b). Annesi (2004) implemented an after-school physical activity program with children ages 9 to 12 years. After assessing for depressed mood, the youths engaged in cardiovascular and resistance exercises three times per week for 12 weeks, or they did not engage in exercise. Annesi (2004) found a significant reduction in depression for the exercise group.

Crews, Lochbaum, and Landers (2004) examined the effects of a physical activity program on the psychological well-being of low-income, Hispanic, children in the fourth grade. A sample of children participated in a 6-week program and were assigned to either an aerobic group involving stationary bicycling, track running, and jumping on a trampoline or a control group that participated in shooting basketballs, walking, and playing foursquare. The authors obtained pre- and posttest depression scores and, at the end of the intervention, the aerobic group reported significantly less depression than the control group. The effect size of −.97 indicated a large impact of exercise on depression in this experimentally based study.

Although the general thrust of the research shows that physical activity is associated with a significant reduction in depression, some maintain that exercise can be a preventive measure, too. Goodwin (2006), for example, studied how effective physical activity is as a coping strategy. In contrast with other strategies that adolescents often use (e.g., substance use, emotional coping, aggressive behavior), Goodwin found that physical activity decreased the likelihood of future depressive episodes. Again, this finding suggests that physical education programs within the schools can be a real benefit in promoting both physical and mental health in youths (Motta, 2018b).

No intervention is universally effective with all groups. Norris, Carroll, and Cochrane (1992) investigated the impact of a 10-week exercise program on the adolescents' psychological well-being. The researchers assigned participants to a high- or moderate-intensity exercise group, or to a flexibility group and determined intensity levels by degree of heart rate elevation (Motta et al., 2012). Pre- and posttest measures revealed no significant reduction in depression scores for any of the groups. It is difficult to know why this finding occurred, but a common issue with many studies is that participants may not have been depressed at the outset of the study. Methodological quality is critical in examining the impact of an intervention. Ideally, researchers should prescreen participants for depression and then randomly assigned them to an exercise or no exercise group. They should take care to ensure that the no exercise group engages in an activity that equalizes the time spent and amount of interpersonal contact so that the only difference between groups is the amount of exercise in which children engage. Pre- and posttest measures should be psychometrically defensible, and it is often desirable to have a follow-up period to see whether intervention effects are maintained over time.

Implications of Using Exercise to Impact Anxiety, Depression, and PTSD in Children and Adolescents

Abundant and ever-increasing evidence shows that exercise can be of significant benefit in reducing adult affective disorders, including PTSD. Hundreds of empirical studies have established the beneficial effects of exercise on adult anxiety and depression, the major components of PTSD. In addition, an increasing number of studies are showing that exercise has direct and beneficial effects on adult PTSD. The emerging research shows that exercise is also of value for adolescents and children. One of the values of physical exercise in reducing negative affect is that it fits within the natural ecology of childhood and adolescent activity. Because physical education classes frequently are available in their schools, children and adolescents view exercise as an integral part of the educational process and part of what it means to be a student in that school system. In contrast, psychotherapy and psychotropic medication are alien to youths (Motta, 2018b).

Children and adolescents, somewhat unlike adults, tend to not pursue therapeutic interventions for issues related to troubling experiences or emotional difficulties (Motta et al., 2012). Indeed, many children who have experienced traumatic events are treatment averse (Dubner & Motta, 1999). However, because including exercise programs into the school setting fits with how children view school, children are less likely to resist exercise than they would traditional psychotherapeutic interventions. It is essential that physical education teachers, school administrators, and school psychologists collaborate on implementation of effective exercise programs in their schools (Motta et al., 2012).

Additional work is needed to develop empirically sound methodologies for investigating the role of exercise in dealing with PTSD and other affective disorders. Clinicians and others have long viewed exercise as of value for the physical well-being of children, adolescents, adults, and seniors. Empirical findings indicate that exercise has beneficial effects on psychological functioning, too (Motta, 2018b). Further research should examine the benefits of exercise as a method of prevention for children and adolescents at risk for internalizing disorders (i.e., troubling emotional states that do not find outward expression).

AEROBIC VERSUS ANAEROBIC EXERCISE: WHICH IS BETTER?

Studies are needed to compare the efficacy of different types of exercise, and additional investigations need to compare exercise with traditional psychotherapeutic interventions (Motta et al., 2012). One of the problems in investigating aerobic versus anaerobic or strength-training exercises is that they are often not mutually exclusive. Strength training can induce an elevation of heart rate, and therefore the separation between aerobic and anaerobic exercise becomes problematic. Current research has weighed heavily in favor of aerobic exercise activity; however, this statement should not be interpreted as meaning that anaerobic exercise is of no value. Some have suggested that the beneficial effects of exercise result from improvements in cardiovascular functioning. Research, however, does not support this position; rather, positive emotional effects are often reported after one session of exercise—long before any healthful physical consequences would be possible. Overall findings point in the direction of any form of vigorous exercise having beneficial psychological effects for reasons that remain unknown.

In a review of studies comparing aerobic and anaerobic exercise, Elkington, Cassar, Nelson, and Levinger (2017) gathered the results of 42 studies that included 2,187 participants. Of those studies, 37 included aerobic exercise; two, resistance exercise; one, a combination of aerobic and resistance; and two compared the effects of acute aerobic exercise with those of acute resistance exercise. The authors found that acute aerobic exercise might ease psychological distress, increase positive well-being, and could help decrease risks of cardiovascular disease. Because of the limited number of studies, though, it was unclear whether aerobic or anaerobic exercise brought about outstanding psychological benefits (Elkington et al., 2017). It was further concluded that obese, overweight, and healthy-weight individuals all benefit from exercise of any kind and that psychological benefits become apparent even after a single exercise session. The previously mentioned Altchiler and Motta (1994) study noted that both aerobic and anaerobic exercise had positive psychological effects. Neither was demonstrably superior to the other.

So, what are we to conclude regarding aerobic and anaerobic exercise? To some extent, the question of which of these two forms of exercise is better is somewhat like the question of which form of relaxation is best. The answer seems to be that the best form of relaxation and the best form of exercise are the kinds that people are more likely to do. If meditation works for an individual as a form of relaxation, then that is best for that person. If brisk walking or jogging suits one better than resistance training or weights, then that is the kind of exercise that a clinician should be prescribe. The available empirical research does not provide clear direction about which form of exercise bestows more psychological health benefits.

Practicing clinicians probably do not trouble themselves with picking through randomized controlled trials of exercise. They know that whatever exercise the client is likely to do is the one they will endorse and support. The research provides no clear direction on which form of exercise is best. It may be that most studies point to aerobic exercise as being beneficial simply because it is easier to quantify and standardize than anaerobic exercise. Clear definitions of aerobic exercise are available, but nonaerobic exercise is not so easily defined, and therefore, the impact of such activity is more difficult to specify. What is known is that exercise beneficially affects emotional states, PTSD, and well-being; therefore, it is a valuable alternative to traditional forms of psychotherapy. The choice of aerobic versus anaerobic activity might also be influenced by the age under consideration. Children and young adolescents might prefer aerobic activity. Many adults might prefer a combination of aerobic and anaerobic, whereas seniors might select aerobic exercise in the form of brisk walking. To repeat: The best exercise is likely to be the one an individual is most likely to continue doing. And, regardless of the nature of the traumatic experience that one has endured, the overall message from the available research is that exercise can significantly reduce the emotional distress associated with such traumas.

SUMMARY

Empirical support shows that exercise is valuable in treating not only PTSD but also the anxiety and depression that accompany this disorder. The available studies are of relatively recent origin and are not numerous. Nevertheless, one sees large effects when exercise is used in treating affective disorders and PTSD in adults, adolescents, children, and seniors. For that reason, a number of clinicians, researchers, and I recommend that exercise be used as a therapeutic adjunct and even as a stand-alone treatment for PTSD, anxiety, and depression. Its ability to enhance well-being and self-esteem are additional benefits.

6

Nature- and Animal-Assisted Therapies for PTSD

A combination of factors may be responsible for the increasing interest in nature- and animal-assisted therapies. Some factors are the sizable numbers of returning military veterans and the inability of the health care and U.S. Department of Veterans Affairs systems to manage such large groups; aversion that many people with posttraumatic stress disorder (PTSD) have to seeking treatment and confronting their problems; desire to avoid medical interventions; effort to minimize the stigma of treatment of trauma disorders; and expense and inconvenience of traditional therapies.

As each name implies, *nature-assisted therapy* (NAT) and *animal-assisted therapy* (AAT) incorporate nature and animals, respectively, within a therapeutic context with a goal of alleviating trauma-related problems. And although these types of therapy may be increasingly popular, researchers are generally uncomfortable with the relative lack of randomized controlled trials (RCTs) for these methods of treatment. Furthermore, clear-cut definitions of what these forms of intervention entail are also lacking. For example,

> NAT is defined as an intervention with the aim to treat, hasten recovery, and/or rehabilitate patients with a disease or a condition of ill health, with the fundamental principle that the therapy involves plants, natural materials, and/or outdoor environments, without any therapeutic involvement of extra human mammals or other living creatures. (Annerstedt & Währborg, 2011, p. 372)

NAT can involve the art and science of plant care and propagation, and the provision of an environment that benefits clients, such as wandering

http://dx.doi.org/10.1037/0000186-007
Alternative Therapies for PTSD: The Science of Mind–Body Treatments, by R. W. Motta

gardens, meditation gardens, and restoration and healing gardens, all of which are not well defined and, for the most part, are relatively lacking in empirical research. Also included within the rubric of NAT are wilderness therapy, outdoor adventure therapy, and *shirin yoku* (Japanese for forest bathing), where physical contact with nature is a critical element. For purposes of treatment, NAT is oriented toward improving psychological, intellectual, social, and physiological outcomes, and outcomes associated with recidivism (Relf, 2005). One can see from the variety of definitions that overwhelming difficulties may hamper systematic investigation of these forms of therapy.

The same holds true for AAT. Studies are available on animals trained to provide a particular service, such as Seeing Eye dogs, or animals trained to work with people with PTSD, such as "service" dogs. Service dogs may shield their handlers from contact with strangers, increase their attention to handlers at times when the handlers seem depressed or withdrawn, and provide other benefits. And animals may function more as pets, providing emotional support; mental health professionals certify some animals specifically as providers of this type of support. In addition, researchers have conducted studies involving dogs (e.g., Paws for Veterans), cats, horses (equine therapy), dolphins, parrots, fish, mice, rats, and guinea pigs (Abdill & Juppé, 2005).

To complicate matters further—not that this is needed—some forms of therapy meld NAT and AAT, including those that involve swimming in tanks with sharks (to overcome fears and gain a sense of control), therapeutic fishing, and animal training and riding in natural environments. Sometimes NAT and AAT are used in combination with traditional cognitive behavior therapy (CBT) and exposure therapy and psychotropic medications. Any effort to disentangle which of these elements is contributing to improvement and by how much is daunting, to say the least. Nevertheless, since the 1990s, traumatized individuals, and especially large numbers of veterans, have pushed for NAT and AAT types of interventions (e.g., O'Haire & Rodriguez, 2018; Poulsen, Stigsdotter, & Refshage, 2015), so one would have to assume that they are of some benefit in alleviating suffering.

TYPES OF NATURE-ASSISTED THERAPY PROGRAMS

The most common types of NAT programs are sustained expedition or base camp models having a duration of 2 to 3 months. Others are trips of about 1 month. The goal of these trips is to develop a greater sense of self-reliance and a more positive view of one's capabilities or *self-efficacy*, if one is to use social-learning terminology (Bandura, 1997). Found in different forms and settings worldwide, adventure therapy programs occur primarily outside but can be carried out effectively indoors. Clinicians use these programs as a primary treatment method or an adjunct to other therapies. Clients engage in activities like rope courses, group games, trust activities, and expeditions into the wilderness. The therapeutic goals frequently include decreasing behavioral problems, such as substance abuse; cultivating psychosocial skills and enhancing psychological resilience; and assisting with internalizing or externalizing psychological problems (Bowen & Neill, 2013).

A number of factors differentiate adventure therapy from other psycho-therapeutic treatment modalities. Adventure therapy programs tend to emphasize learning by experience through awareness of or interaction with nature. These programs also use perceived risk to create positive stressors and increase the client's arousal, focus on positive change through problem solving, provide meaningful engagement in the adventures, and offer group-based interventions that frequently are fundamental to the experience and treatment methodology (Bowen & Neill, 2013).

By exposing participants to individual and group challenges, one benefit is that they will deal with such exposure effectively and subsequently see improvement in their sense of self-esteem. Another benefit is physical activity, which Chapter 5 in this volume showed had a significant positive impact on negative emotional states, such as anxiety, depression, and PTSD. Another health-promoting factor, according to some perspectives, is that by being within a green, natural, living environment, one becomes part of it. One draws closer to the earth and nature, which are self-sustaining and homeostatic, and therefore one also resonates with self-sustaining energy (Williams, 2017).

Some wilderness therapy programs are designed for troubled teens and expected to be therapeutic, meaning they employ highly trained clinical personnel to accompany the youths. Other wilderness programs are geared toward older adolescents and young adults. Some are more in line with a base camp model and tend to have a military and endurance emphasis rather than a therapeutic focus. Personnel employed by this model with a military-endurance emphasis may be former military or corrections officers who focus more on participants' developing an enhanced sense of self-capability to endure stress. And then other wilderness programs are entirely unstructured and designed to simply encourage people in general to experience and benefit from nature (Bowen & Neill, 2013). Clearly, these models have a good deal of overlap.

It has been proposed that humans have a natural affiliation with and attraction to nature. Wilson (1984), an entomologist, used the term *biophilia* to describe this phenomenon, although social psychologist Erich Fromm coined the term to describe a passionate love of life and living things ("Biophilia Hypothesis," n.d.). Biophilia is one of the reasons that people wish to build their homes near trees or water, and why they visit zoos more than they attend all of professional sports combined. Natural environments tend to present people with a sense of being away from life's stressors, which they experience as mentally fatiguing. Engaging with nature is stress reducing and restorative. One can only speculate why human beings find nature engaging. Perhaps it is our evolutionary past in which we were much closer to and dependent on nature favored those who most benefited from this interaction, and we are the products of that evolutionary history. We are also part of nature, and from that perspective, why wouldn't we feel a sense of attunement and benefit from engaging in the essence of who we are?

Rozak (1995) has been credited with the term *ecopsychology* to describe the relationship between human beings and nature through ecological and psychological principles. Many names have referenced ecopsychology, including Gaia psychology, psychoecology, environmental psychology, green psychology, global therapy, green therapy, nature-based psychotherapy, and sylvan therapy. The central premise tying these terms together is that although in today's world we are increasingly distanced from nature through our technological and social advances, our deep neurological structure has been formed through interaction with the natural environment. We human beings and the natural environment are inseparable. In damaging the environment, we are doing damage to ourselves. By making our environment increasingly toxic, we are threatening our own survival. Separation from nature may be akin to separation from the source of our own essence.

Researchers (e.g., Donovan et al., 2013) have proposed and demonstrated that engagement with nature improves one's sense of peace, improves interpersonal relationship, and promotes well-being. Therefore, clinicians attempt to move therapy outside and away from formal offices. Similarly, gardening has been associated with stress reduction, resiliency following stressful experiences, and beneficial changes in cortisol levels. Improvements in self-efficacy across age groups and increased attentiveness also has been demonstrated. Those who are engaged in horticultural activities and in wilderness adventures show perceived alleviation of pain, restored social connectedness, joy, and reductions in negative rumination.

Abundant available evidence indicates that NAT has beneficial psychological and physical effects. Its value in dealing with PTSD is that it is nonintrusive. It does not require a traumatized individual to revisit and reprocess traumatic images and memories. For this reason, NAT is far less likely to elicit the avoidance response that plagues so much of the psychotherapeutic attempts to manage PTSD. One of the difficulties in conducting research in NAT is that many varieties of environments and situations might be considered "natural." Thus, one sees studies examining wilderness adventures, gardening, outdoor exercise and socialization, horticultural activities in general, life close to nature, and so on. The inability to specify and agree on a definition of *nature* or *natural* impedes methodologically controlled research. Nevertheless, the overall thrust of the research (e.g., Poulsen et al., 2015) suggests that nature in and of itself can have beneficial effects on humanity and that it might be fruitful to integrate nature into standard treatments of psychological distress. Clinicians are well advised to encourage traumatized clients to spend time in natural environments, even if the only impact of this interaction is the reduction of negative emotional states and attitudes.

TYPES OF ANIMAL-ASSISTED THERAPY PROGRAMS

Therapists traditionally trained in areas such as CBT, psychodynamic therapy, relational therapies, or psychopharmacological forms of treatment typically are not exposed to training in AAT or NAT. It is unusual for therapists to use animals in treatment even though they may have pets of their own and have a kinship with animals. Why might this be? Therapist training programs often center around a theoretical orientation that focuses on how psychopathology develops and treatments usually follow from these theoretical views. Animals simply do not fit into standard models of training and treatment. It is also possible that therapists may be hesitant to introduce an animal into the therapy session for fear of what the client's reaction might be. Clients may have an aversion to animals, be allergic to them, or have a number of other reasons for feeling uncomfortable with animals in the therapeutic setting. And yet, considerable literature attests to the therapeutic value of AAT (e.g., Eggiman, 2006; Parish-Plass, 2008; Sobo, Eng, & Kassity-Krich, 2006), even in treating PTSD (e.g., Rodriguez, Ryan, Rowan, & Foy, 1996). The range of animal types used as therapeutic adjuncts is wide and includes dogs, horses, potbellied pigs, cats, birds, hamsters, dolphins, reptiles, llamas, and sharks. The animals can be either trained for specific therapeutic purposes or untrained.

The use of animals as therapeutic adjuncts is really nothing new. Sigmund Freud often included his chow, Jofi, in psychoanalytic sessions. He observed that many of his clients' long-hidden fears and verbalizations did not trouble the dog; thus, their anxiety was reduced and a discussion of a client's difficulties was facilitated (Beck, 2010). Florence Nightingale (1969) valued the presence of pets in the treatment of ill individuals. In the early 1900s, St. Elizabeth's Hospital in Washington, DC, found value in pet–human bonding in terms of improving recovery (Huck & Burke, 2019). In 1980, University of Pennsylvania researchers found that clients with pets lived longer after heart attacks than those without pets (Abdill & Juppé, 2005). Many hospitals today encourage interaction of clients and animals, and some health facilities regularly bring in animals so that clients can interact with them.

The range of human afflictions for which animal assistance can be of benefit is wide and includes anxiety disorders, major depressive disorder, inadequate personality disorder, attention-deficit/hyperactivity disorder, autism spectrum disorder, PTSD, Alzheimer's disease and other dementias, high blood pressure, and reactions to abuse in its various forms. One can only speculate why animals may be therapeutically beneficial. Perhaps it is because they are incapable of the scheming, strategizing, and planning that is so readily available to those with well-developed cerebral cortices and frontal lobes. As such, their response to humans is refreshingly honest, accepting, and nonjudgmental, which is particularly beneficial to those whose traumatic experiences have left them avoidant of interpersonal involvements and as having deficiencies in trust. Most animals used in therapy can form bonds with humans, and because of the unconditional acceptance that animals display, people perceive them as nonthreatening and validating to their interactions with them. Even animals that don't seem to readily form bonds, such as fish and reptiles, can nevertheless enhance one's sense of efficacy through appropriate and effective care and management of them. Regardless of the reasons for the beneficial effects of animals as therapeutic adjuncts for a variety of conditions, it seems reasonable to incorporate them into therapy, particularly for those whose traumatic experiences have left them avoidant of any form of therapy that deals directly with the traumatic experiences, such as prolonged exposure therapies and CBT.

Before delving into research on AAT, I should note that animals are of therapeutic benefit when available as pets and as formally trained therapy animals. When using a therapy animal, it is accompanied by a handler or partner. Therapy sessions usually do not exceed 2 hours to avoid tiring the animal. Approximately 10,000 animal and handler partnerships exist in the 50 states and internationally. Pet Partners, formerly the Delta Society, is one of the primary organizations that certifies therapy animals, and provides this commonly accepted definition of *animal-assisted therapy:*

> Animal-assisted therapy is a goal-oriented, planned, structured, and documented therapeutic intervention directed by health and human service providers as part of their profession. A wide variety of disciplines may incorporate AAT. Possible practitioners could include physicians, occupational therapists, physical therapists, certified therapeutic recreation specialists, nurses, social workers, speech therapists, or mental health professionals. (Pet Partners, n.d., "Industry Terms," para. 2)

CASE EXAMPLE: USING ANIMAL THERAPY WITH A TRAUMATIZED ADOLESCENT

Tommy was an 11-year-old boy when I saw him. His parents were so eager to get help for their withdrawn son that they drove each week from their home in Connecticut to my office in Long Island, New York. They were desperate. Their son was once an extroverted, athletic, verbal, and highly sociable youngster, and was also a strong student. One summer, his parents provided him with sailing lessons at a school conveniently located on Long Island Sound. By the end of summer and the end of the sailing lessons, Tommy was a changed person. He had become moody and withdrawn, and he no longer desired to take sailing lessons. It turns out that an older man—his sailing instructor—had sexually abused him. When the parents finally pried this information out of Tommy, the outcome was the incarceration of the sailing instructor, but that action did little to help Tommy.

Tommy was particularly withdrawn in my presence. He was alone in a room with an older man for a therapy session. What could be scarier for this boy? And, yet, working out his feelings and processing them with an older man seemed just what he needed. I must admit that we made little progress during the first few sessions. And then, one day, Tommy's mother called me and said that her son asked if he could bring his pet hamster to the session. I agreed even though, frankly, I felt it a bit odd to be sharing a therapy session with, what to me, was a rodent. Well, I learned a lesson during the next session when Tommy arrived with his hamster in a cage outfitted with an exercise wheel. He was noticeably more relaxed. He had his familiar friend with him, and it had a noticeably calming effect on him. His newfound lack of anxiety allowed for a freer exchange of information and helped Tommy unload the details of the burden he was carrying. After a few additional sessions, his mood began to lift, and he started going out with friends. Previously he had hidden in his room and was accompanied only by his computer. Now, he even went so far as to suggest that he might be interested in sailing again, although to my knowledge, he did not do so. Overall, the hamster that Tommy brought into his sessions may have served as a protection for him. It was a familiar friend that helped Tommy confront his awful secrets in detail and to thereby move forward. The hamster was, in many ways, a confidant and support that made being in therapy easier to manage. The message was clear to me: Just as Freud's dog, Jofi, had helped his clients during those early explorations of psychoanalysis, Tommy's hamster helped him in the explorations of his trauma and in his eventual healing. The hamster in itself did not produce an immediate "cure." What it did, it seems, is to help create an environment that facilitated change. It made the hard work of therapy a little more manageable.

In any therapeutic setting, it is difficult to know what it is that brings about beneficial changes. Was it Tommy's hamster that served as a catalyst for change, or would this change have come about anyway? Was the change because his loving parents were willing to go out of their way to seek help for their son and to believe him when he reported to them that his sailing instructor had touched him inappropriately? Could the change have resulted from working with an older male therapist whose emotional nurturance and support helped counter the belief that men could not be trusted? There is no way of knowing for certain, but it seemed clear that the presence of Tommy's pet hamster produced a certain calmness or easing of anxiety in this boy, which may have set the stage for his willingness to begin the process of change. It is odd to have a hamster as a cotherapist, but if that what is needed, most therapists would welcome it.

EMPIRICAL STUDIES

In keeping with the theme of this book, I attempt to review some of the empirical work that has been done to evaluate NAT and AAT. Overall, there does appear to be a measurable benefit from nature- and animal-assisted interventions, although the actual measurable effects do not seem overwhelming. One of the major problems in evaluating any new form of intervention is what has become known as the *file-drawer problem*: When positive results are found, they are published. When no results or negative results are found, they are placed in one's files and do not make it into print. The cumulative effect is a biased positive evaluation of the research because of the abundance of positive published outcomes. Although one might say the file-drawer problem can be relevant to any form of investigation, including the types of traditional therapies, it is especially problematic in the areas of NAT and AAT because of the few high-quality studies on which to rely and, therefore, a relative lack of objective criteria for evaluating outcomes.

Value of the Outdoors

Numerous empirical studies show that simply being outdoors in nature has beneficial psychological effects. I review these studies in detail later in this chapter. Participants engaging in social interactions and physical activity rate these activities as significantly more revitalizing when conducted in outdoor environments than indoors. The studies also show substantial increases in vitality on validated measures when individuals engage with natural environments. Study participants rate aquatic environments as being the most restorative, and rural environments (e.g., hills, woodlands, forests) as being the second most restorative. Urban environments are rated as significantly lower on scores of health restoration. To quote Florence Williams (2017) from her book *The Nature Fix*, "Go outside, often, sometimes in wild places. Bring friends or not. Breathe" (p. 254).

When using a computerized measure of sustained attention designed to mentally fatigue participants, studies show that when participants are then called on to view nature scenes, there was a measurable improvement in attention on returning to the computerized task. Viewing nature scenes has led to significant reductions in negative affect and increases in positive affect on psychometrically valid measures, as well as a slowing of heart rate on electrocardiogram measures. These results hold even when viewing simulated nature scenes in video presentations in addition to being in actual natural environments. Such results show promise in working with those who have anxiety, depression, and PTSD. Similarly, viewing nature videos results in lowered blood pressure as measured by pulse transit time and skin conductance response, which measure the sweat reaction to stress. Viewing nature scenes leads to significantly greater reduction in these physiological stress measures when compared with viewing urban scenes.

Are Randomized Controlled Trials Possible or Desirable With Nature- or Animal-Assisted Therapy?

The idea behind an RCT is that the researcher makes careful efforts to isolate the influence of a variable or variables of interest. In the pharmaceutical world, what typically takes place is that a group of individuals are randomly assigned to conditions in such a way that there is no way of knowing which group received the medication under investigation and which group received a substance that is expected to have no effect, usually a placebo. Often those administering the medications, in addition to those receiving the medications, do not know which group is getting the active medication and which, the placebo. This is the *double-blind procedure*.

Even in tightly controlled designs, such as double-blind randomized controlled studies, researchers may have problems isolating effects. Take, for example, the impact of *expectancy*: People expecting they might get better from a medication or placebo may actually feel better. Extensive literature shows that placebos have some impact on improving health, so a placebo is not the inert intervention that the experimenter may have intended. In addition, study participants may desire to please the experimenters, which can translate into the belief of, and reporting of, improvements in health whether or not they exist. Then, consider the *volunteer effect*: Those who volunteer for studies may have characteristics that differ from the population as a whole, which can make generalization from the experimental world to the "real world" a questionable leap. Some have convincingly argued that results of experiments are only generalizable to experimental situations and those who participate in them: "What works in research settings may not be the same as what works in practice" (Waddell & Godderis, 2005, p. 60). It seems that the more precisely the experimenter obtains a tight, valid experiment, the less ecologically valid, or generalizable, are the findings. So, although RCTs may be the best approach researchers have of validating interventions, it is extremely difficult to obtain incontrovertible findings even with this approach. Now, if this is true in the seemingly tightly controlled world of pharmaceutical research, what can we say about NAT or AAT research? Are RCTs possible or desirable?

Gabrielsen, Fernee, Aasen, and Eskedal (2016) set out to explore the possibility of using RCTs in wilderness and adventure therapy. They randomly assigned a group of emotionally troubled adolescents to either the adventure group or the treatment as usual (TAU) group. Their study was not an actual RCT but, rather, an exploration of the possibilities of conducting RCT's with adventure interventions. What the researchers came to realize is that those who were not assigned to the adventure group but who had volunteered to participate in the study were likely to be highly troubled by their assignment to the TAU group. These youths typically had experienced abusive or neglectful childhoods and, as a result, had a negativistic view of life and a diminished sense of self. Being assigned to the TAU group would only further validate their negative views of themselves and their environments. Consequently, any comparison between the groups would be influenced by the nature of the design itself. One would no longer be comparing youths who participated in the outdoor adventure to controls but, rather, to a TAU group that was now further embittered and negative. The between-group comparisons would be invalid because the TAU group had been negatively altered by the experimental procedures.

Another problem recognized by Gabrielsen et al. (2016) was that no one could accurately define TAU because treatments vary among individuals and within the same individual over time. TAU can even be no treatment at all. A further problem they identified involved ethics. The question arose as to whether it is ethical to move forward with a study in which needy, youthful participants are denied potentially beneficial interventions for the sake of experimental validity.

One possibility considered by the researchers was to have participants serve as their own control such that they would first be informed of a multimonth adventure study but not allowed to participate for a period equivalent to that of the adventure experience. In this way, a control group would be formed of the participants themselves, thereby eliminating certain threats to validity. The problem, though, is with the waiting period. Assessments during the waiting period might negatively impact the youths in that they would see that nothing exciting follows the testing, and that might come across as another example of unmet promises.

Ultimately Gabrielsen et al. (2016) decided to have a "lead-in" period in which assessments were taken as part of the youngster's normal routine without providing the expectation of an adventure study. Once they had obtained data from the lead-in period, they might compare those data to data from the adventure study that was subsequently initiated at posttest and follow-up. Although the authors proposed this approach, they did not carry it out, which gives the reader an idea of why RCTs may be few and far between in NAT and AAT types of interventions. They are difficult to effectively run.

Furthermore, outdoor, nature-based programs are identified by a number of different names as are NAT programs in general, which complicates research. For example, Bowen and Neill (2013) delineated these outdoor programs: "wilderness therapy, wilderness adventure therapy, wilderness experience programs, bush adventure therapy, adventure-based counselling, outdoor adventure intervention, therapeutic camping, and outdoor behavioral health-care" (p. 28). These experiences most often occur in natural settings and are said to engage individuals emotionally and cognitively while they engage in physical activity. The goal of these programs is to serve as an adjunct to traditional psychotherapy or to be a stand-alone intervention for emotionally and behaviorally troubled individuals.

Meta-Analyses of Outdoor Nature Programs

The actual meta-analyses conducted of outdoor programs include within their statistical compilations the different types of outdoor programs just described by Bowen and Neill (2013). What they have in common is that they are oriented toward the development of healthy cognitive and behavioral functioning through activity within the natural environment.

Bowen and Neill (2013) conducted a meta-analysis of these programs. Their analysis combined the results of 197 studies of adventure therapy participant outcomes and examined more than 2,900 effect sizes of different measures. The overall rounded effect size for adventure therapy in their investigation was moderate (.50). That effect size was slightly lower than effect sizes reported for meta-analysis of individual psychotherapy (.68) but indicated a meaningful and statistically significant impact. For no-treatment comparisons included in the study, the effect size was .08; for alternative nonoutdoor programs, it was .16. Both effect sizes were considered small or minimal. The authors found little change during the lead-in period (a process advocated earlier) or assessment period in which there was no program (.09), or in the follow-up periods (.03) for adventure therapy. Those results showed long-term maintenance of the short-term gains. In seven out of the eight outcome categories, the outcomes of short-term adventure therapy were significant: The clinical and self-concept measures had the strongest effects. The effects for spirituality/morality were the smallest. Bowen and Neill found a positive relationship with participant age: Older participants benefited to a greater degree. They also discovered during their meta-analysis that since the 1960s, the research literature on adventure therapy studies has been reporting larger effects. As a result, research is proceeding to strongly support the effectiveness of outdoor programs.

Publication bias analyses indicated that the Bowen and Neill (2013) study might have slightly underestimated true effects. As Bowen and Neill stated in the abstract to their article,

> overall, the findings provide the most robust meta-analysis of the effects of adventure therapy to date. Thus, an effect size of approximately .5 is suggested as a benchmark for adventure therapy programs, although this should be adjusted according to the age group. (p. 28)

In the area of clinical research, an effect size of .5 is considered respectable, and researchers are generally satisfied with this level of impact. It is reasonable to state then that adventure therapy programs are meaningful and effective interventions for ameliorating social, behavioral, and emotional problems, and can certainly be considered to be of value to those suffering from trauma.

Neill (2003) commented that only about 7% of adventure therapy programs use measures one can use in meta-analytic studies. Therefore, it is difficult to get a handle on the actual overall effectiveness of these programs. The effect sizes could be greater or less than those reported in meta-analyses. Neill also noted that a small effect size can be impressive if, for example, what one is attempting to change does not readily yield to external influence (e.g., dysfunctional behavior) or if the outcome, like recidivism, is highly valued. Similarly, large effect sizes might not necessarily mean that there is therapeutic value related to the goals and aims of treatment (e.g., physical fitness). Clearly, statistical outcomes must be combined with clinical judgments to obtain a more accurate picture of the value of NAT.

In Neill's (2003) review of meta-analytic studies involving approximately 12,000 participants, overall effect size was .3 to .4 (respectable) on typically measured outcomes like self-confidence and self-esteem, and those results seemed to increase in follow-up periods. The most effective outdoor education programs were ones with adult participants, that were longer, and that were conducted by established organizations, such as Outward Bound.

Because some effect sizes ran from about .21 to .34 in the studies reviewed by Neill (2003), one needs to stay away from blanket claims of effectiveness. Rather, I and undoubtedly others recommend that a finer grained analysis be done on particular programs—for particular populations—seeking specific outcomes. A need exists for analyses of program length, client problems, sequencing of activities, facilitation style, and the like. For example, the reviewed studies show a variation in effect sizes ranging from 1.05 (large effect size) for clinical scales of outdoor and adventure-based programs to .24 (small effect size) for measures of well-being. Nevertheless, the overall conclusion of these varied analyses is that these outdoor therapy programs have a significant positive impact.

Annerstedt and Währborg (2011) attempted a synthesis of both controlled and observational studies of NAT while also including three meta-analyses. In addition to the meta-analyses were six well-controlled studies and 29 studies of low- to moderate-evidence grade. Among the latter group of studies, 26 of the 29 reported health improvements because of NAT. The authors stated,

> This review gives at hand that a rather small but reliable evidence base support the effectiveness and appropriateness of NAT as a relevant resource for public health. Significant improvements were found for varied outcomes in diverse diagnoses, spanning from obesity to schizophrenia. (p. 371)

One can see from the available research that NAT is a beneficial "alternative" therapy for a wide variety of conditions. Many traumatized and emotionally and behaviorally troubled individuals have gravitated toward NAT, not because of empirical evidence of its value but simply because it seems to ease their distress.

Empirical Evidence for Animal-Assisted Therapy: Trained Service Dogs for Veterans With PTSD

Many of the CBT interventions can be effective for those who are able to endure them. The problem is that the majority of traumatized veterans simply find CBT and exposure-based interventions too much to bear because such procedures cause intolerable levels of anxiety. This is where trained service dogs can be of substantial benefit. Service dogs differ from assisted therapy animals (e.g., rabbits, horses, dogs), emotional support animals, and pets in that they are trained specifically to engage in behaviors directed to the needs of those with psychological difficulties (O'Haire & Rodriguez, 2018). Military veterans who have returned from combat environments and who have PTSD comprise one of the major available groups of individuals who fit this description.

Service dogs lessen the impact of PTSD among veterans by promoting a sense of safety, independence, and confidence. They are able to engage in behaviors that mitigate the effect of nightmares, panic reactions, depressive withdrawal, and alienation from the environment typically seen in PTSD. These service dogs have been associated with improvements in socialization on the part of veterans, reductions in panic reactions, and improvements in sleep. Yet one of the problems with these observations is a relative lack of empirical support from controlled studies. General consensus seems to be that the presence of trained support animals, and even untrained ones, can be of real benefit, and veterans appear to willingly volunteer to be engaged with support animals. Although, again, the relative lack of hard data to support this consensus is a problem. It appears that the positive feelings that animals invoke in many people lead to the belief that their presence is beneficial, but belief and evidence are quite different, and empirical studies are needed to support these beliefs.

One such study that did provide evidence of the value of trained service dogs was conducted by O'Haire and Rodriguez (2018) and published in the prestigious *Journal of Consulting and Clinical Psychology* of the American Psychological Association. This journal is known for its high standards and methodological rigor in the research it publishes. In the study, O'Haire and Rodriguez compared a national sample of veterans who had applied for a service dog with veterans who already had one. Participants had to have an honorable discharge or be currently in service, have a documented diagnosis of PTSD from a health professional using psychometrically sound measures, have no current or past history of substance abuse, and have met other exclusion criteria. The final sample included 66 wait-list controls and 75 who had been with a service dog for an average of 1.6 years. Service dogs were primarily Labrador retrievers, golden retrievers, and mixed breeds. A professional training organization, K9s for Warriors, provided the dogs. Once participants were placed with a service dog, they attended a training class for 3 weeks. They lived in dormitories at the dog training site and attended daily scheduled activities. The participants trained the dogs to respond to specific commands, but, more importantly, the dogs' training included learning how to be alert to and react to a client's anxiety and agitation to help avert panic attacks. The dogs also were trained to wake their charges from nightmares, lean against the veteran or stand to form a barrier between the veteran and others so to lessen anxiety associated with violations of personal space, retrieve and remind veterans to take prescribed medication, and allow veterans to lean on the dog for stability.

The O'Haire and Rodriguez (2018) study produced comparisons over time for those who had a service dog and comparisons between wait-list participants and those who had dogs assigned to them. Those who had dogs and those who did not have them were not restricted in any way from the usual care—TAU—that they may have or have not been receiving for managing their PTSD.

Results indicated significant reductions in PTSD symptoms for those in the service dog group over time and during a follow-up period. These reductions were not seen in the wait-list controls. Although these reductions were shown to be substantial, they did not produce reductions large enough for veterans to now meet the criterion set for no PTSD on a standardized PTSD measure. The magnitudes of the reductions in PTSD scores, however, were shown to be comparable with those seen in traditionally accepted treatments, such as CBT. In addition, participants with service dogs exhibited significantly lower depression symptomology with large effect sizes and had improved quality of life compared with those without dogs (O'Haire & Rodriguez, 2018).

In comparison with controls, those with service dogs showed significantly greater ability to engage in social activities, had lower social isolation, and lower rates of absenteeism from work because of health issues. "This pragmatic, longitudinal effectiveness trial has provided initial evidence that, compared with usual care alone, military members and veterans with trained service dogs show lower PTSD symptomology, reduced depression, and increased social participation" (O'Haire & Rodriguez, 2018, p. 183). No perfect studies exist, including this one. However, this trial does provide fairly convincing empirical evidence for value of using service dogs in treating PTSD. The dogs appear to evoke significantly less avoidance in comparison with traditional psycho-therapeutic approaches that emphasize confrontation of one's fears. That veterans volunteer to be partnered with a service dog speaks volumes for this form of intervention.

An analysis of the benefits and challenges of using service dogs for veterans with PTSD was carried out by Yarborough, Stumbo, Yarborough, Owen-Smith, and Green (2018). Their study involved 41 veterans and their dogs. Intensive interviews revealed numerous benefits to those having a service dog, such as these examples:

- Alerting to reduce hypervigilance: The dog rests its head on the veteran's foot, and whenever anyone approaches, it raises its head to alert the veteran that someone is coming.

- Waking from nightmares: When the veteran yells out in the middle of the night, the dog puts its cold nose on the veteran's neck to wake the veteran and prevent further distress.

- Nudging: When the dog senses that the veteran is going into a dissociative state, it pushes against the veteran to move them out of that state.

- Physical and emotional connection: Many traumatized veterans feel emotionally numb and distant from others. Service dogs tend to demand attention and desire contact, which helps the veteran reduce the tendency to withdraw.

- Dog-related responsibilities help activate veterans: Many of those with PTSD have withdrawn from society. They fear the environment because the combat environment was so aversive and dangerous. Dogs force the veteran to get out of bed, feed and care for the animal, and brush him and interact with the animal. All of these activities mitigate the inclination to pull back and be inactive.

- Medication reduction: Owing to the decrease in stress level brought about by being associated with a dog, reports indicate a lessening of the need for blood pressure medication, sleeping pills, and antianxiety and antidepressant medications. I have noticed this outcome in my practice and in the trauma clinic I direct.

All of the preceding benefits did not come about without challenges. Some of these challenges were finding a suitable match between veteran and specific animal, going through training and having to learn to work with the dog, adjusting to a new life with a dog continuously present, experiencing delayed veteran–dog bonding, inviting unwelcome public attention, and having beliefs of increased stigma because of the presence of a service dog. However, the overall conclusion of the study was that "veterans with PTSD experienced several benefits and a few substantial challenges to using service dogs as therapeutic agents to manage PTSD" (Yarborough et al., 2018, p. 123).

Empirical Evidence for Equine-Assisted Interventions

I admit that well controlled empirical studies of the value of horses used for the purpose of stress reduction are few and far between; however, empirically defensible studies are emerging. In one such study (Lanning, Wilson, Woelk, & Beaujean, 2018), 89 military service members diagnosed with PTSD were randomly assigned to an 8-week therapeutic horseback riding (THR) group or to a comparison group. The THR condition consisted of weekly 90-minute sessions, and study participants shared a meal before each equine session. The first 4 weeks included riding and horsemanship exercises. Participants also named a person who knew them well, such as a significant other or family member, who could provide another source of data other than those from self-report measures. For reasons that could not be clearly identified, horseback riding was effective in reducing PTSD and depression to a clinically significant degree, even when those veterans had suffered from PTSD for decades and had attempted many other forms of psychotherapy and medication.

In a similar study carried out by Johnson et al. (2018), 29 military service members with PTSD were randomized to a wait-list control or 6-week THR program. The authors designed the study to assess whether THR would result in a decrease in PTSD symptoms, increase in coping self-efficacy, emotional regulation, and a decrease in social and emotional loneliness. Significant reductions in PTSD were found on standardized measures after 3 weeks, with even greater reductions at 6 weeks. The loneliness, self-efficacy, and emotional regulations measures either did not show significant reductions or moved in a direction opposite to what the authors had expected. The overall conclusion of this well-controlled study was that THR may be a clinically effective intervention for alleviating PTSD symptoms among military personnel.

Another empirical study was conducted involving children and horses (Pendry, Smith, & Roeter, 2014). This investigation attempted to move away from whatever weakness are associated with self-reported measures of psychological improvement by focusing on cortisol measures. The authors randomly assigned children referred by school counselors and children recruited from the community to a wait-list control condition ($n = 60$) or a condition involving interaction with horses ($n = 53$). The group assigned to a condition involving interaction with horses participated in a series of once-a-week, 90-minute sessions of activities facilitated by horses for a period of 11 weeks. Over 2 consecutive days at pretest, the researchers collected six samples of salivary cortisol from the participants in their homes; at posttest, they collected another set of six samples. According to Lupien, McEwen, Gunnar, and Heim (2009), lower basal cortisol levels may constitute a protective influence against the development of psychopathology. In general, lower cortisol levels are associated with stress reduction.

Among the horsemanship activities in which children engaged were mounted and unmounted activities, observing human–equine interactions, observing horse behavior, engaging in the management of the horses (e.g., grooming), walking the horses, riding, and engaging in personal and group reflection (Pendry et al., 2014). These activities also could be carried out with ponies, miniature horses, donkeys, and mules. Those in the equine condition showed lower afternoon cortisol levels and lower hourly cortisol concentration levels compared with wait-list controls. The strength of the Pendry et al. study is that it relied on measures that are difficult to alter. The alteration or changing of scores on measures can result from participants' desire to be a "good" subject and comply with the experimenter. Cortisol levels represent a far more objective measure than self-report measures. But, again, no study is perfect, and one could argue that there were multiple influences on the children in addition to the horses (e.g., social interaction, learning new skills). One could also argue that no one-to-one relationship existed between cortisol levels and stress or pathology. Nevertheless, the results of this study do show statistically significant reductions in cortisol, and cortisol is commonly seen as elevated in response to stress.

An additional benefit of being with horses, and this benefit can certainly apply to any traumatized individual, is that this union trains one to be mindful (see Chapter 4, this volume, for a discussion on the benefits of mindfulness in treating trauma):

> Before we meet the horse, before we even enter the barn, we need to learn how to stay mindful, to be aware of how we are feeling and what we are experiencing in the present moment. Horses live in the here and now; it is the basis of their serenity and survival. Being with them in an invitation to join them in their world. (Buzel, 2016, p. 3)

According to Buzel (2016), being congruent and having your feelings and behaviors match is essential in one's interaction with horses. When a mismatch occurs, when one is pretending to feel a certain emotion, the horse will sense this disjunction and react with uncertainty and confusion, and it will have difficulty connecting with the handler. Sometimes, traumatized veterans who are at a loss to describe their emotions can find serenity in the reactions of a horse that accepts them nonjudgmentally for who they are.

STRENGTH OF EMPIRICAL SUPPORT

It is considerably difficult to conduct well-controlled empirical studies of NATs, and for this reason, the scientific support for this form of intervention is not strong but is nevertheless somewhat compelling. Meta-analyses involving thousands of individuals show moderate effect sizes at about .3 to .5, which are considered to be respectable, and suggest that NAT is of value in treating trauma-related disorders. AATs fare better in terms of garnering scientific support, but not many RCTs exist to rely upon. Traumatized individuals, both military and nonmilitary, who have participated in controlled studies have benefited emotionally and socially from interacting with animals, and have even shown improvements in the biochemical domain as revealed by reduced cortisol levels. The use of natural environments and animals can be considered a viable therapeutic adjunct in treating PTSD.

SUMMARY

It seems clear from available studies that immersion in natural environments and engagement with animals can have significant psychological and physical benefits. Consider that the average person checks their cell phone 1,500 times a week; the typical teen sends 3,000 texts a month; and that the majority of us spend well more than 90% of our time in houses, buildings, and cars (Williams, 2017). And future trends appear to show a movement toward living in cities and away from nature. These trends also show increased levels of isolation, depression, and suicide. Also consider the growing body of empirical research revealing that nature and animals can beneficially impact those with PTSD and other disorders, and even help those who are not so afflicted but are simply burdened by the stresses and strains of modern living. Natural environments and engagement with animals lower blood pressure, anxiety, depression, and cortisol levels. These effects occur even in environments that would be surprising. For example, traumatized veterans who swim with sharks develop a sense of tranquility as a result in being in water. Furthermore, they develop a sense of mastery when they manage their fear of sharks.

Spending time in natural environments and with animals may seem an unusual intervention for traumatized individuals. But, increasingly, this is what they crave. These same traumatized people often have an aversion to exposure-based psychotherapeutic treatments even though these forms of intervention can be highly effective for those who are able to endure them. It is almost as if their traumatized bodies and minds inherently know what is good for them and that the farther they move from their evolutionary beginnings that included nature and animals, the farther they become estranged from themselves. As an alternative intervention, or as an adjunct to traditional psychotherapeutic approaches, nature and animals can be valuable resources for clinicians, who should certainly add them to the therapeutic toolbox. The "gut" positive reactions that many have for nature and animals are increasingly supported by empirical evidence. NAT and AAT have shown themselves to be of value in reducing the pain of PTSD and associated psychological disorders.

7

Acupuncture for PTSD

Many people simply do not know what to make of acupuncture. The process is seen as alien and outside the realm of traditional Western medicine. It uses peculiar terminology and procedures. It is often viewed as lacking in a sound scientific basis, and if it is considered to be of any real value, it might be used for the alleviation of pain for those inclined to try unorthodox methods. Recent research suggests that acupuncture can be of benefit in treating psychological problems, such as posttraumatic stress disorder (PTSD). This research begs the question: How could the placement of small needles under the skin do anything other than be painful, annoying, and anxiety producing, especially for the many who fear needles and other forms of injection? In addition, few clinicians and psychotherapists are trained and have certification in the technique, so consideration of its use would require an outside referral. Training often involves 200 to 300 hours of acupuncture experience for those with medical degrees (Eisenberg et al., 2002), or 2,000 to 3,000 hours in an accredited acupuncture master's degree program (Synovitz & Larson, 2013). Most states also require acupuncture students to pass a board exam. Outside referrals are commonly done when nonmedically trained clinicians refer clients for psychotropic medication, but it is far less common—perhaps even unheard of—to refer out for acupuncture in cases involving psychological distress and PTSD.

Those inclined toward skepticism find an easy target in acupuncture. The process is said to be based on alteration of the energy flow of *qi*, a life force, to produce balance between the two opposing forces of yin and yang, the

http://dx.doi.org/10.1037/0000186-008
Alternative Therapies for PTSD: The Science of Mind–Body Treatments, by R. W. Motta

existence of meridians or energy channels along which qi flows. No part of this process has been validated according to traditional Western medicine and science. Some claim that the location of the placement of the needles does not alter the reported pain-reducing effects of treatment. Because of the approximately 2,000 established needle sites, considerable variability exists in needle placement. Others claim that if there is any real benefit to acupuncture, it is the well-known placebo effect, and needle placement has little impact in and of itself.

WHERE IS THE EVIDENCE?

Substantial evidence points to the effectiveness of acupuncture in the alleviation of both physical and mental distress. I review the empirical evidence in this section. Many researchers and clinicians, however, discount this evidence simply because of an inability to understand the mechanisms by which acupuncture works. It is almost as if no amount of evidence will convince these skeptics. Before examining the evidence for and against acupuncture, let's develop a perspective on the topic by comparing Eastern and Western medicine. Eastern medicine makes no clear distinction between body and soul. Their unity is known as *mind-soul,* a concept akin to Pert's (1999) idea of *bodymind,* which suggests that our acceptance of the quasi-independent entities of body and mind is misguided. They are a dynamic unity, and one is not affected in the absence of the other. Within the concept of mind-soul, psychogenic and physical disorders are understood as conditions caused by the abnormal flow of qi and an imbalance of yin and yang. The mechanisms that regulate qi are not well understood by either Eastern or Western Medicine, and Western medicine is the more doubting. Many Western researchers and physicians skeptically maintain that acupuncture's impact is little more than a placebo effect but do not seem equally doubtful about commonly accepted placebo effects in Western medical procedures. One such accepted medical procedure is called *meniscectomy,* an arthroscopic process whose efficacy is unquestioningly accepted by most physicians.

Meniscectomy is a surgical procedure that approximately 700,000 people a year receive to ease pain resulting from a tear in the cartilage (i.e., the meniscus) that cushions the knee (Jaslow, 2013). *The New England Journal of Medicine,* however, reports that a Finnish study (Sihvonen et al., 2013) showed that the practice of performing arthroscopic meniscectomy for degenerative meniscal tears may be misguided. In a typical procedure, the surgeon inserts a small camera into the knee and removes torn pieces of cartilage using tools such as a mechanized shaver. This procedure costs approximately $4 billion annually, yet according to the study's authors (Sihvonen et al., 2013), over-the-counter pain medication, exercise, and rest may be just as effective as the surgery. In short, meniscectomy may be little more than placebo.

In the Sihvonen et al. (2013) study, researchers assigned patients at random to either have the arthroscopic meniscectomy or undergo a sham procedure that resembles that surgical process but uses a bladeless mechanized shaver against the outside of the knee (Jaslow, 2013). The sham group received the same amount of time in the operating and recovery rooms, as well as the same amount of postoperative care as those who underwent surgery. Although both groups showed improvements in symptoms from their baseline questionnaires, no significant differences in pain relief were found between the real surgery group and the sham group (Jaslow, 2013).

To some extent, the results of the sham meniscectomy bear a similarity to the results of some acupuncture procedures in that the underlying mechanisms of change are unclear. The difference is that meniscectomy is no more effective than placebo interventions, whereas many studies show acupuncture to be more effective than placebo. Just as the real pain-reducing mechanism of meniscectomy may be rest, exercise, over-the-counter pain medication, icing, and so forth, the real pain-reducing mechanism of acupuncture may be something other than the unblocking of qi. At this point, it is unclear why acupuncture works despite evidence for its efficacy.

BRIEF HISTORY OF ACUPUNCTURE AND ITS UTILITY

The first documented history of acupuncture as an organized system of diagnosis and treatment appeared approximately 2,500 years ago in China and is based on the traditional teachings of Taoism, which emphasizes harmony between humans and their world, and balance of the opposing forces of yin and yang. By the early 19th century, travelers to China began introducing acupuncture and Chinese medicine to the West. In France, acupuncturists focused much of their attention to the sites in the ear and their effect on distant body functions. Acupuncture started to become popular in the United States in the 1970s and was given a boost by President Richard Nixon's trip to China. Since then, guidelines have been developed in the United States to govern the use of acupuncture and organized societies of acupuncture have been established (Watson, n.d.). According to a 2002 survey, approximately 8.2 million Americans have tried acupuncture, and this number had risen to 14.01 million by 2007, and those Americans were using acupuncture primarily to ease pain (Su & Li, 2011).

With each passing year, acupuncture has gained in popularity and respectability. A 2004 study by Berman et al. in the *Annals of Internal Medicine* found that acupuncture produced significant reduction in pain resulting from osteoarthritis. A 2006 Mayo Clinic study by Martin, Sletten, Williams, and Berger found significant improvement in fibromyalgia, which causes fatigue, joint stiffness and muscle pain. Chemotherapy-induced nausea was found to be significantly reduced by acupuncture, as reported in a 2000 study by Shen et al. in the *Journal of the American Medical Association*. Studies by Zhang et al. (2011) in the *Fertility and Sterility Journal* reported increased pregnancy rates in women who received acupuncture while undergoing in-vitro fertilization procedures. Bladder-control problems were significantly reduced by acupuncture, as reported in *Obstetrics and Gynecology* by Emmons and Otto (2005).

World Health Organization's View of Acupuncture

The World Health Organization (WHO; 2002) took on the task of exploring the validity and utility of acupuncture given its wide usage especially in Eastern nations and many other parts of the world. The review covered various forms of acupuncture, including *moxibustion* (herbs burned on or over the skin); traditional body needling; *electric acupuncture*, involving electrical current supplied to needles; microsystem acupuncture (e.g., face, ear, scalp, hand); and *acupressure*, pressure applied by the practitioner to selected sites. WHO reviewed a number of well-controlled studies, and some produced indisputable scientific evidence that, in certain situations, acupuncture is more effective than placebo treatments. The results in other studies were less clear: Acupuncture relieves about 55% to 85% of chronic pain, which compares well with the proportion of analgesic drugs (in 70% of cases, morphine is helpful) and 30% to 35% placebo (e.g., Pomeranz, 1989; WHO, 2002). According to WHO (2002), scientific research has revealed specific actions of acupuncture, such as bringing on pain relief, regulating bodily functions, and helping the body fight infection.

Different acupuncture points and manipulations may produce a bidirectional effect (WHO, 2002). For example, acupuncture lowers blood pressure in patients with hypertension and increases it in those with hypotension. In patients with muscle weakness in the intestines or with spastic colitis, acupuncture, observed by X-ray, restores intestinal motility (WHO, 2002). Therefore, the overall impact of acupuncture is to normalize body processes through mobilization of the organism's own healing potential. It facilitates balance or equilibrium within the organism.

In many of the published trials WHO (2002) reviewed, providers had executed sham acupuncture by needling at "incorrect, theoretically irrelevant sites" (p. 7). Positive results are evidence that carrying out *genuine* acupuncture according to established procedures is more effective than *sham* acupuncture. The negative results from trials in which genuine and sham acupuncture were both considerably therapeutically effective and had no significant difference between them does not mean that genuine acupuncture is ineffective (WHO, 2002). If sham acupuncture significantly reduces pain, for example, this finding might be interpreted as evidence that sites other than the genuine acupuncture might also be effective.

The WHO (2002) report lists a wide range of conditions "for which acupuncture has been proved" (p. 33). A sample includes lower back pain, nausea and vomiting, neck pain, facial pain, headache, hypertension and hypotension, morning sickness, and unfavorable reactions to chemotherapy or radiotherapy. Among the emotional disorders that have been significantly improved is depression resulting from psychogenic factors or stroke. Other studies have demonstrated significant reductions in anxiety, which is of relevance to the issue of PTSD because depression and anxiety are among the more prominent symptoms of this disorder. PTSD was formerly categorized as an anxiety disorder in the fourth edition of the *Diagnostic and Statistical Manual of Mental Disorders* (*DSM–IV*; American Psychiatric Association, 1994) before being listed among the trauma-related disorders in the current *DSM* (fifth ed. [*DSM–5*]; American Psychiatric Association, 2013). Following some preparatory comments, let us look at evidence for the efficacy of acupuncture for trauma-related disorders.

Can Acupuncture Be Used as a Treatment for Trauma Disorders?

A number of psychological and physical processes are involved with PTSD aside from the impact of having experienced a traumatic event or events. Some of these are internal processes, such as anxiety and depression, and many are of a physiological nature. Given that acupuncture is a physical procedure, it stands to reason that acupuncture might have an impact on PTSD because many physical processes are associated with the disorder. Some of these internal and physical processes include

- Comorbidity: Approximately 50% to 60% of those with PTSD have major depressive disorder (Hollifield, 2011). Anxiety is also a major component in the vast majority of cases. Acupuncture appears to have an impact on anxiety and depression.

- Physiologic disorders: Those with PTSD show higher rates of cardiovascular disease, arthritis, hypertension, autoimmune disorders, fibromyalgia, psoriasis, irritable bowel syndrome, diabetes, and others (Kimerling, 2004). Acupuncture has been used successfully with many of these disorders.

- The central nervous system: Neuroimaging studies (e.g., Alfermann & Stoll, 2005; Shin et al., 2004) of those with PTSD show increased activation of the amygdala during reexperiencing of trauma and a suppression or lack of cortical activation especially noted by suppression of activity in the medial prefrontal cortex and anterior cingulate cortex. These neurological centers and their activity, or lack of activity, are what appears to be the neurophysiological basis of the failure to recover from traumatic experiences (i.e., activation of the amygdala and suppression of the cortical controls). The amygdala is associated with fear responding unmitigated by reason. Among the activities of the cortex are reason, organization, and problem-solving. Acupuncture reportedly results in suppression of the overactivity of the amygdala and activation of the prefrontal cortex (Lanius, Bluhm, Lanius, & Pain, 2006).

- Hypothalamic–pituitary–adrenal (HPA) axis: The interaction and feedback of these centers control reactions to stress and mediate the general adaptation syndrome. Dysregulation of this axis occurs in PTSD and results in a lack of regulation of cortisol, elevation of specific neurotransmitters and hormones, and sensitization of receptors. Acupuncture is said to bring about a healthy regulation and balancing of the HPA axis (Yehuda & LeDoux, 2007).

- The autonomic nervous system: Studies show activation of the sympathetic nervous system (i.e., fight–flight–freeze response) when one encounters a traumatic experience. The sympathetic response far exceeds that shown in response to nontraumatic stressors. Few studies report on parasympathetic system activity in response to trauma. Acupuncture is reported to quell overactivity of the sympathetic nervous system (Blanchard et al., 1996).

- Inflammation: PTSD is associated with low-grade inflammatory markers. Inflammation is recognized to accelerate atherosclerosis, encourage insulin resistance, alter pain responsiveness, and accompany infection. Acupuncture reduces pain and is said to subdue the inflammatory response (Rohleder & Karl, 2006).

Hollifield (2011), following a careful assessment of modern Western medicine and Chinese medicine stated, "Conceptual, clinical, and biological data support the potential efficacy of acupuncture for PTSD" (p. 775). Both forms of medicine identify individual variables and external stressors as causal to the development of PTSD. "In both traditions, the field will benefit from identifying core clinical and biological features that are more specific to PTSD [than other disorders]" (p. 776). To date, Western medicine finds interventions such as those derived from cognitive behavior therapy (CBT) to be effective in treating PTSD. In Chinese medicine, acupuncture has been a mainstay in the treatment of this and many other disorders.

Randomized Controlled Trial Involving Acupuncture in Treatment of PTSD

Throughout this review of alternative methods of treating PTSD, I have made an effort to detail empirical findings, especially those derived from randomized controlled trials (RCTs). Clinicians and researchers often trash new and alternative methods of therapy; for this reason, it is important to detail the hard evidence or data for these alternative methods. In writing these words, I admit that I have been one of those who have repudiated "new" approaches, such as eye-movement desensitization and reprocessing (EMDR), which I covered in Chapter 2. EMDR has subsequently clawed its way into respectability because prominent researchers were no longer able to deny its place in the compendium of highly effective psychotherapeutic interventions for PTSD. EMDR is now considered to be a validated and empirically supported treatment by many professional organizations including the Society of Clinical Psychology (Division 12) of the American Psychological Association (APA Presidential Task Force on Evidence-Based Practice, 2006). Nevertheless, despite the evidence for EMDR or acupuncture, a large number of skeptics remain with perhaps the majority within the professional and research communities.

Unfortunately, acupuncture has not attained a similar level of respectability as EMDR for dealing with PTSD, despite supportive evidence. It is unclear why this is the case. Perhaps it is because one requires intensive training to develop competence, and few clinicians or researchers have such training. Its lack of acceptance also could be because of the alien terminology it uses, such as liver fire, heart/yin blood deficiency, kidney yang/qi deficiency, and heart shen disturbance. Needle placements have strange locations, including ST 36, HT 7, BL 20, and GV 14. No one other than those with specific training would have any idea what these sites refer to. Clearly RCTs are needed so that acupuncture can attain some level of acceptance as a treatment for PTSD.

One such RCT was conducted by Hollifield, Sinclair-Lian, Warner, and Hammerschlag (2007). Their study not only evaluated the efficacy of acupuncture for PTSD and related problems but also compared it with CBT and a wait-list control (WLC). The acupuncture intervention alternated between 11 needles in the front of the body and 14 needles in the back during 1-hour sessions, twice per week, for 12 weeks. Standard acupuncture points were used for all participants in this group, and a few flexibly prescribed points could be added to meet individual characteristics. Solid needles were used with manipulation (i.e., no electrical stimulation was used). The intervention was compared with Group CBT that ran for 2-hour sessions for 12 weeks. CBT consisted of a number of elements, including psychoeducation, behavioral activation, activity planning, cognitive restructuring, imagery rehearsal, exposure, and desensitization. Thus, the amount of intervention was the same between treatment groups and equivalent to 24 hours. The WLC did not receive treatment but did provide data.

The study was designed to randomly assign volunteer participants to groups using a computer-based random number generator. The research coordinator who analyzed the data had no idea which participant was in which group but was simply provided with data obtained from acupuncture, CBT, and WLC groups and conducted the statistical analyses. This is a standard "blind" procedure designed to eliminate or at least minimize experimenter bias effects.

Both acupuncture and CBT showed significant reductions in PTSD symptoms from pre- to posttreatment, and large effect sizes exceeding 1.0 (.2 is considered small; .5, medium; and .8, large; Cohen, 1987). Both interventions exceeded the WLC, which showed only minimal changes. Improvements were maintained in a 3-month follow-up. The authors also found significant reductions in anxiety and depression in the acupuncture and CBT conditions, and these reductions were statistically equivalent between treatment groups (Hollifield et al., 2007). This study is important in that it shows acupuncture to have an impact on PTSD equivalent to CBT, and yet, in the treatment of PTSD, no actual psychotherapy was provided.

Despite the well-controlled nature of the study by Hollifield et al. (2007), no investigation is without its flaws. One could argue that acupuncture was compared with Group CBT, but CBT is traditionally conducted individually. Theoretically, this nontraditional way of conducting CBT could have reduced the impact of CBT, making it more equal to acupuncture in its impact. One might argue that the volunteers for this study were highly motivated and do not represent the typical sufferer of PTSD who is less inclined to volunteer for anything. Many other critiques could be leveled at this RCT and many critiques also could be found with any study on any topic. To get a fairer picture, one must look at overall trends in the outcomes of studies. Even this approach can be critiqued in that overall trends reflect what is published, not what may be unpublished and is in the "file drawer." At the very least, studies are out there that show that acupuncture reduces PTSD anxiety and depression, and this evidence is important to clinicians.

WHY USE A PROCEDURE THAT MOST CLINICIANS DON'T KNOW?

No one can provide accurate numbers, but clinicians would agree that the majority of those who have been traumatized or have PTSD do not seek psychotherapeutic intervention. Traditional methods of treatment almost always involve some discussion of dealing with or revisiting the traumatic experience and the associated negativism of the experience. Doing so evokes a high level of anxiety. The level of anxiety is so high that it creates an aversion to and avoidance of traditional treatment of any kind. Even therapists find the process of repeated confronting unpleasant and typically avoid therapeutic approaches that involve reexposure to trauma material. These difficulties on the part of clients and clinicians are what moves those suffering from trauma experiences in the direction of interventions such as acupuncture, yoga, meditation, and exercise which place minimal emphasis on actual traumatic experiences. If clients can find relief of emotional pain in procedures that don't involve reactivation of that pain, that is the direction in which they often go, and that is also the direction in which caring therapists might wish to direct their clients.

A good deal of research—despite the skepticism of many—shows that acupuncture is effective in relieving pain, and emerging empirical studies are providing evidence for its utility with troubling emotional conditions, such as depression, anxiety, and PTSD. It is certainly not the treatment for everyone with troubling emotional disorders, but if psychotherapy-averse PTSD sufferers can find relief of distress from the unusual process of having needles inserted into the skin, or by engaging in yoga, meditation, or some other alternative therapy, who are we to question this? Although acupuncture may not be a first choice for most clinicians, it is certainly an option to consider when more traditional approaches have failed.

DESPITE RANDOMIZED CONTROLLED TRIALS, DO HARD SCIENTIFIC DATA EXIST ON THE VALIDITY OF ACUPUNCTURE?

If one examines many of the studies on the effectiveness of interventions for PTSD and related symptoms, it appears that almost all of the them use self-report measures, regardless of whether we clinicians are evaluating CBT, exposure, yoga, and just about any other kind of therapeutic intervention. Even in acupuncture in which the focus may be on the alleviation of pain, we depend on our client to tell us the level of discomfort. A self-report measure, which relies on the respondent to provide information on their condition, can be influenced by that participant's belief that they have been affected by the treatment, by the desire to please the experimenter, by the influence of the procedure (like the use of needles), and by many other factors. A PTSD sufferer may report that they experience migraines at a level of 7 or higher on a 10-point scale. That same individual might complete reliable and valid paper-and-pencil measures of PTSD, anxiety, and depression, and although these measures maybe psychometrically sound, they continue to rely entirely on what the PTSD sufferer reports. So, when one considers the impact of acupuncture, it would be of considerable value to know whether any objective information goes beyond self-report. Such a study has been conducted using acupuncture for carpal tunnel syndrome.

Carpal tunnel syndrome is a painful wrist condition resulting from the entrapment and compression of the median nerve. The nerve entrapment can cause pain, weakness, numbness, and sometimes loss of sensation of hot and cold. Some studies show actual evidence of deterioration of muscles, ligament, and tendons. A 2015 study by Ding and Shen reported in the *Journal of Clinical and Experimental Medicine* focused on the gathering of objective data from sufferers of carpal tunnel syndrome who underwent acupuncture. The procedure involved the application of acupuncture needles along standard meridians. Every 10 minutes during 30-minute sessions, the acupuncturist stimulated the needles using manual acupuncture techniques, and study participants received acupuncture once each day of the week over a 6-week period (Ding & Shen, 2015). In total, the study had 30 acupuncture treatment sessions. Moxibustion was also applied to heat the acupuncture points, called *acupoints*. The moxibustion process involved the application of heat from the burning of herbs in a metal box held over the needle insertion points. To say that this is not traditional Western medical practice is the height of understatement.

Aside from verbal reports of reduced pain and actual increased mobility, the study (Ding & Shen, 2015) also performed a large number of objective electrical conduction tests. They assessed the postintervention client status by procedures that they called distal motor latency of the median nerve, thumb-to-wrist sensory conduction velocity, and other objective electrophysiological tests. The authors confirmed improvements in nerve transmission by testing the velocity of motor conduction, potential of both sensory nerve action and compound muscle action, the velocity of sensory conduction, and distal motor latency. Using high-resolution ultrasound imaging, Ding and Shen (2015) demonstrated notable improvements in the areas of transverse carpal ligament and median nerve transection. Another study published in *Neural Regeneration Research* (He et al., 2015) demonstrated that acupuncture causes injured lower and upper limb motor nerves to repair. Electromyography confirms that acupuncture significantly improves motor nerve conduction velocity and amplitude, and also promotes functional nerve repair.

What the wide variety of electrophysiological and ultrasound tests indicated in the Ding and Shen (2015) study was significant improvement in carpal tunnel syndrome and other types of nerve injuries as measured by objective methods. The study also found that acupuncture results in significant improvements that go beyond the critiques, such as placebo effects, power of suggestion, experimenter bias, and others. Extraordinary claims (improvement through needling) are said to require extraordinary measures (electrophysiological and ultrasound assessments). It appears that acupuncture does work in controlling carpal tunnel pain and other kinds of neuropathology and that the hard data provided are difficult to dispute. I write this fully realizing that true skeptics will be able to find fault with any study and raise disputes no matter what. For example, participants in the aforementioned studies must be highly motivated to deal with 30 sessions of acupuncture. Perhaps this motivation translated into actual healing as a number of nonacupuncture-related studies have shown. No one study is definitive without multiple replications. Some doubters of the efficacy of acupuncture indicate that the beneficial effects are quite small and that studies using "real" acupuncture sites do not differ much from those that use sham site (i.e., those in which needles are randomly placed). Yes, skeptics always have a lot to chew on regardless of study quality and objectivity of measures.

SHAM VERSUS GENUINE ACUPUNCTURE

The issue of genuine versus sham acupuncture was addressed in a meta-analysis of 29 RCTs by Vickers of the Memorial Sloan Cancer Center. Published in the *Archives of Internal Medicine*, the study (Vickers et al., 2012) came to the following conclusion:

> Acupuncture is effective for the treatment of chronic pain and is therefore a reasonable referral option. Significant differences between true and sham acupuncture indicate that acupuncture is more than a placebo. However, these differences are relatively modest, suggesting that factors in addition to the specific effects of needling are impotent contributors to the therapeutic effects of acupuncture. (p. 1444)

Sham acupuncture included a procedure without needles, such as using a detuned laser or deactivated electrical stimulation; acupuncture needles that were inserted superficially; or sham acupuncture instruments having retractable needles that didn't penetrate the skin (MacPherson et al., 2017). The average effect of acupuncture in the this metanalytic study was .5, which is considered to be a medium effects size and also is considered to be respectable and acceptable in studies assessing therapeutic effectiveness. This small difference between genuine and sham acupuncture suggests that "[unknown] factors in addition to the specific effects of needling are important contributors to therapeutic effects" (Vickers et al., 2012, p. 1414). Vickers et al. (2012) concluded that rather than concern themselves with the issue of the relative efficacy of genuine or sham acupuncture, health care providers would do better determining whether to refer clients to this procedure when pain is the issue. The authors found that such a referral is warranted based on the data.

Another study of sham versus genuine acupuncture did not find a difference between the two procedures in a study of 100 clients with fibromyalgia (Assefi et al., 2005). The treatments were for 12 weeks with either an acupuncture program specifically designed to treat fibromyalgia or one of three sham treatments: acupuncture unrelated to fibromyalgia, needle insertion at non-acupoint locations, or noninsertive-simulated acupuncture. Clients were blinded to what treatment procedure they were receiving. For all they knew, they were receiving a credible acupuncture procedure for their condition. The good news of the study was that the procedures had an overall beneficial effect. The believer in the importance of specific acupuncture points or acupoints based on qi and energy-transferring meridians would be troubled by the non-support of these concepts by this study. Whether acupuncture is releasing hormones, altering neurochemistry, impacting and rewiring neural circuitry or some other process, or doing a combination of processes is unclear. What is clear is that many people suffering from physical illness, emotional distress, or both do find relief in acupuncture and sometimes choose it over more traditional and sometimes less effective traditional Western medicine procedures. It appears that the specific approaches used in acupuncture are of less importance than the use of acupuncture itself.

Before moving on to other areas in which acupuncture has shown its value, let's keep in mind the earlier cited studies showing that certain arthroscopic knee surgeries were no more effective in alleviating pain than sham arthroscopic procedures. Knowing this information seems to have had little impact on the number of people who seek out this surgery. One may not know for sure why those in the sham surgery condition reported pain reductions similar to those in the real surgery condition, just as one may not know why those in genuine and sham acupuncture showed similar levels of improvement. It is possible that the body has a natural tendency to move toward health if provided with the right conditions. Traditional Western medicine and traditional Eastern medicine may activate the conditions needed to facilitate a return to health even though the explanatory constructs of these two traditions differ markedly. There seems little justification for doubting the outcomes of one tradition and extolling the virtues of the other when both seem to produce healthy adaptations. Recall that people accepted the beneficial effects of aspirin for many years without having any idea how it worked. And yet it does work.

ACUPUNCTURE INTERVENTIONS FOR PTSD SYMPTOMS

Acupuncture has traditionally been seen as an effective intervention for physical pain. More recent research findings have shown that it can also be effective in treating PTSD and symptoms associated with that disorder. One of the primary symptoms of PTSD is anxiety, and acupuncture has been found to be a useful intervention for anxiety.

Acupuncture as a Treatment for Anxiety

For most of its existence, PTSD has been categorized as an anxiety disorder in earlier iterations of the *DSM* (e.g., *DSM–IV*). It has now attained its own place among the trauma related disorders in *DSM–5*. What this means is that anxiety, along with its cohabitant, depression, are among the more prominent features of PTSD. It is the disturbingly high levels of anxiety that prevent those who are traumatized from seeking psychotherapeutic treatment. Traditional treatments massively elevate anxiety because these interventions require a reprocessing of and reexposure to traumatic memories. The aversion to revisiting trauma memories is what opens the door to acupuncture as an alternative treatment.

Errington-Evans (2012) reviewed numerous studies on the use of acupuncture for anxiety, including those representing Western and Eastern medicine traditions; they also included animal studies. This author noted that in addition to PTSD, anxiety is the main ingredient in panic disorder, agoraphobia, social phobia, obsessive-compulsive disorder, acute stress disorder, generalized anxiety disorder, and others. The individual studies that Errington-Evans reviewed varied in the nature of the samples (e.g., volunteers, clients, students, community samples, animals). Studies also varied in their use of randomization, degree of blinding, use of controls, and sample sizes, which varied from four to 240, but overall large sample size studies were used. Animal studies used such methods as sucrose intake in which subjects with matched food intakes differed in their consumption of sucrose solution, and this difference was associated with higher levels of anxiety. In addition, the animal studies offered the opportunity to apply immunohistochemistry directly to brain tissue for markers of stress-induced depression or anxiety, or both, so the researchers could examine the biochemical effects of acupuncture. To summarize the findings, Errington-Evans (2012) stated, "The quality of the research pertaining to the use of acupuncture in the treatment of anxiety disorders varies greatly. Results are almost universally positive" (p. 280) despite the poor quality of the reporting.

If acupuncture is indeed useful in treating anxiety problems, as the Errington-Evans (2012) review purports, then it is important to provide some picture of the nature of this intervention. In the studies reviewed, the number of acupoints used varied from one to 34; three was the most common. The number of sessions per week varied from one to 7; 3 was the mode. Total number of sessions ranged from one to 40; 10 was the most used. And session duration ranged from 30 seconds to 1 hour; ½ hour was the most common. Acupoints used were both those based on traditional Eastern medicine guidelines and alternatives that some authors refer to as sham acupoints.

Errington-Evans (2012) reported that acupuncture as a treatment of anxiety is progressing slowly and in an uncoordinated fashion. In general, the methodological reporting is poor and the research is frequently lacking rationale for point selection. The author stated that evidence shows that acupuncture compares favorably to CBT, which is the common intervention for treating anxiety disorders. The setting in which acupuncture takes place and the methods used are generally less stressful and therefore more willingly sought out than CBT. This researcher, along with many others who have investigated the effects of acupuncture, stated that other researchers must make it a priority to provide consistent, evidence-based recommendations on the dosages required so that acupuncture will be therapeutically effective.

The wide range of quality in the research studies of acupuncture, along with the equally wide variation in sampling and methods, makes acupuncture an easy target for those who are uncomfortable with this mode of treatment. However, it seems that if acupuncture were ineffective in treating anxiety, it would not have such worldwide acceptance from those afflicted with this disorder. Undoubtedly, a file-drawer problem (see the definition in Chapter 6) is in these studies, whereby null or negative results are hidden away and positive results are published. However, it is unlikely that the typical person suffering from anxiety spends their time reviewing research studies. These suffering individuals rely on word-of-mouth recommendations from friends, family, and professionals. And they appear to be deriving some benefit from acupuncture, as the popularity of this approach to treatment shows.

Acupuncture as a Treatment for Depression

Anxiety and depression are probably the two most prominent features of PTSD. The two disturbances are commonly found together, and some would argue that where one exists, the other is likely to be present. The overall weight of evidence shows a 50% overlap such that when anxiety is present, depression is also present at least half the time. However, in disorders such as PTSD, it is unusual to find anxiety without depression.

WHO stood behind acupuncture as a treatment for depression. That acupuncture may be effective in treating depression as well as emotional, neurological, and physical disorders continues to leave open the question of the mechanism by which these beneficial effects occur. The bottom line is that, like the positive effects of exercise, no one knows for sure why these effects occur.

A study by Sun et al. (2013) set two goals. The first was to compare acupuncture with the psychotropic medication Prozac (fluoxetine), which is a serotonin reuptake inhibitor, as treatments for depression. The second goal was to move beyond self-report as a source of study data by also measuring glial-cell-derived neurotrophic factor (GDNF), which plays a role in the pathogenesis of depressive disorder and may be a biomarker for damage to nerve cells. The study had three conditions, two of which involved the use of different methods of acupuncture. The first condition used acupuncture sites guided by clinical perspectives (i.e., those that had proven most useful in clinical practice). The second acupuncture method was based on acupoints frequently used for depressive disorder as prescribed by methods used in China. These two acupuncture conditions were compared with a third group that received fluoxetine.

The samples comprised volunteers who responded to a public announcement of a study involving the treatment of depression and who were between the ages of 18 and 70. Sun et al. (2013) obtained pretest measures using the Hamilton Depression Rating Scale (Hamilton, 1960), a 5-point scale ranging from 0 (*not present*) to 4 (*severe*) and also involved blood and urine testing. The acupuncture included electrical stimulation in place of manual manipulation. Participants received acupuncture treatments five times per week for 6 weeks. At the same time, participants in the fluoxetine group were treated with oral fluoxetine (20 mg/day) for 6 weeks. The researchers evaluated each client's symptoms at the beginning of the study, and at 2, 4, and 6 weeks of treatment. They measured serum GDNF before and after 6 weeks of treatment. There were 20 clients in the first acupuncture group, 16 in the traditional Chinese medicine acupuncture group, and 25 in the fluoxetine group. Groups did not differ in terms of age, gender, weight, height, body mass index, age of onset duration, and other demographic factors, or on initial Hamilton Depression Rating Scale (Hamilton, 1960) scores or GDNF levels.

Results indicated that the two acupuncture groups "showed great improvement" (more than 90% improved), whereas the fluoxetine group had 84% improvement. These percentages are impressive by any measure, and perhaps eyebrow raising. The acupuncture groups were statistically more effective in symptom reduction than the medication group. After 6 weeks, GDNF levels increased in all groups compared with baseline. One of the differences that stood out was that the acupuncture groups responded more quickly with depression reductions than the fluoxetine group. It is not an uncommon observation to see some delay in the lifting of depression symptoms with selective serotonin reuptake inhibitors. Sun et al. (2013) noted that GDNF exerts a neuroprotective effect and is a potent factor for the health of dopaminergic neurons. The results were found to be consistent with reports of increased GDNF with a variety of antidepression treatments.

The study of the utility of acupuncture with emotional disorders such as anxiety, depression, and PTSD is in the early stages of development. The research on medical conditions and acupuncture has a longer history, and far more studies exist.

CASE EXAMPLE: PRESCRIBING ACUPUNCTURE FOR ANXIETY AND DEPRESSION FROM COMPLEX PTSD

Raymond is a highly competent 62-year-old construction supervisor who is entrusted with virtually all decisions regarding the construction of various buildings in Manhattan, New York. He has the necessary licenses and certifications, and he can juggle the personnel, supplies, equipment needs, and the paperwork needed to complete a construction project. Despite his competence, he has a spotty employment history that often involves leaving a construction project because of some interpersonal conflict with project owners. He is easily offended by anything other than glowing praise for his work. In addition, Raymond suffers from generalized anxiety disorder and major depressive disorder for which he is receiving psychotropic medication and psychotherapy. In therapy, it became clear that much of Raymond's emotional difficulties and sensitivities resulted from childhood sexual abuse at the hands of his father. He is classified as having complex PTSD because of this abuse. The abuse is one of Raymond's demons, and it has altered his life in every way. He is thin skinned and moody, and he suffers panic attacks. Raymond distrusts relationships so has never married, although he has been in a relationship with a girlfriend for 20 years. He harbors a fear that he too could be a child sexual abuser, even though the fear has no basis. Although able to see the connection between his sexual abuse and his emotional dysfunctions and distrust of others, Raymond's anxiety and depression have persisted.

Raymond reports that from the time he was 3 until he was 14, he was forced to engage in masturbatory activities, and that on many occasions, his father would pin him down while thrusting against him. Raymond would struggle to free himself but was never successful in doing so. When asked which of these two forms of abuse disturbed him the most, unquestionably, being pinned was the most frustrating and anxiety provoking, and it elicited the most anger on his part. The inability to escape and being trapped are hallmarks in the development of PTSD. Raymond has kept this demon of sexual abuse under wraps and has not shared it with family members. He fantasizes about confronting his father but is no longer able to because his tormentor has passed away.

Raymond's second demon has been a persistent head and neck pain that has lasted for years. These relentless, stabbing pains resulted from a fall from a construction ladder that led to his smacking his head onto concrete. Although he continued working for 2 weeks after the fall, he subsequently underwent a magnetic resonance imaging procedure. While awaiting the results of the scan, a doctor appeared and informed Raymond that he was going to the hospital in an ambulance because the procedure had revealed bleeding on the left side of his brain, evidence of a large subdural hematoma. Surgery involved lifting off a segment of his skull and relieving the compression of the brain caused by the buildup of blood between the brain and skull. Although the surgery was successful in alleviating the pressure, the pain persisted. Raymond visited many health care providers representing various specialties and was prescribed a large number of painkillers, but the pain continued. Raymond then made an appointment with an acupuncturist who had helped an employee on one of the construction sites who had also sustained an injury. He was reluctant to make the appointment because he believed acupuncture was nonsensical, but the pain motivated him to do so.

The acupuncturist explained that something was preventing Raymond from overcoming his pain and that the body and mind normally had a tendency to heal themselves. Acupuncture was presented as a means of allowing these natural healing processes to take place. Raymond visited the acupuncturist for weekly session over a period of 3 months, and he began to experience a reduction in head and neck pain after the first session in which a series of needles were placed into the skin in the back of his neck. This result this took Raymond by surprise; he had expected that this procedure, like all the others he had tried, would also fail.

The acupuncture appears to have worked, and as a result, Raymond's physical pain demon no longer torments him. Strangely, acupuncture appears to have also facilitated an emotional healing, thus weakening his emotional demon. Raymond reports that his depression appears to have lost its intensity, and his anxieties also have been reduced since he started the acupuncture treatments. These reductions of negative emotion have facilitated a willingness to more openly discuss and process his childhood sexual abuse; they also have allowed him to begin to be more trustful of others. It was stunning to hear that he decided to move in with his girlfriend. He had never considered making such a commitment in the past.

In clinical situations such as this, it is difficult to disentangle what therapeutic element or elements led to positive changes. Psychotherapy, psychotropic medication, and acupuncture were involved as were numerous pain medications taken over time. However, it appears that psychological and physical progress were at a standstill up to the point at which acupuncture was introduced. The interpretation of the acupuncturist is that the blockage to mind-soul healing was lifted by acupuncture. Most importantly, Raymond sees acupuncture as having triggered a movement toward health and serving as a catalyst for change that had not been achieved by the other interventions he had received. It is cases such as Raymond's that support the use of acupuncture as an adjunct to or as a stand-alone treatment for many physical and emotional ailments.

STRENGTH AND LIMITATIONS OF ACUPUNCTURE FOR PTSD AND ASSOCIATED DISORDERS

The primary strength of acupuncture from the perspective of those suffering from PTSD is that it does not require the client to revisit their traumatic experiences. The extremely high levels of anxiety that this reexposure causes often results in clients' fleeing therapy. Acupuncture does not require repeated confrontation with trauma experiences. One simply sits through a needle insertion process or similar procedure, and assuming they have no emotional reaction to the methods, there should experience little elevation of anxiety and a fair chance of symptom improvement. From the researcher's perspective, the accumulation of hard data from electrophysiological, imaging, and bio-chemical studies bodes well for increasing acceptance of acupuncture.

The limitations of acupuncture include its inconvenience. Two of the studies described earlier required clients to endure five sessions per week for 6 weeks. Thirty sessions of at least a half an hour each is a good deal to ask of anyone. In today's time-pressured society, visiting a therapist for 30 consecutive sessions is highly unlikely to take place. Even when the average number of sessions is 10, as reported by Errington-Evans (2012), this is still demand-ing, especially when multiple acupuncture sessions each week are required. Another limitation is cost. Many insurance carriers will not pay for acupuncture for PTSD or other emotional disorders, and the out of pocket expenses can be prohibitive. The unusual nature of acupuncture is another potential limitation that might keep clients away. It looks nothing like traditional medicine or psychotherapy.

Considering both strengths and limitations, acupuncture undoubtedly has provided, and will provide, relief to at least some of those suffering from PTSD, anxiety, depression, and physical disorders. For this reason, it is a viable alter-native to traditional treatment approaches.

SUMMARY

The empirical support for acupuncture as a treatment for PTSD, anxiety, depression, and pain-related problems is substantial, although probably not as compelling as that shown for EMDR as a PTSD treatment. Acupuncture has become popular in the United States since the 1970s but has a 2,500-year history. WHO supports it as a treatment for physical and various psychological disorders. A number of scientific studies show actual physiological changes in addition to psychological improvements as a result of acupuncture. Acupunc-ture does have respectable empirical support, but it requires specialized training, and for this reason, it is not an easily accessible alternative treatment for PTSD, despite its scientific merit.

8

Emotional Freedom Techniques for PTSD

Emotional freedom techniques (EFT) are a form of intervention linked to acupuncture in that they focus on energy, energy blockages, meridians, and methods designed to facilitate body energy flow to facilitate health. Whereas the primary method of acupuncture involves needles, the focus of EFT is on physically tapping or rubbing areas of the body associated with hypothesized energy-carrying meridian end points. EFT is based on the position that ill health, whether physical or emotional, results from energy blockages and imbalances in meridians, and that tapping helps releases the blockages and balances the energies. By balancing these energies, the body and mind are enabled to engage is self-healing.

EFT, which has been used in the treatment of a wide array of disorders, evokes a colorful and often vitriolic back-and-forth in the literature. On the one hand, sites like Wikipedia describe it with such pejorative descriptors as "pseudoscience" and "placebo effect," and suggest EFT is ineffective, pre-scientific, and essentially nonsensical ("Emotional Freedom Techniques," n.d.). On the other hand, publications of numerous well-controlled studies have appeared in respected, peer-reviewed medical and psychological journals that attest to its effectiveness. The counterresponse to these supportive findings is that the studies are flawed and of little scientific merit.

It is important to consider for a moment what happened in the history of the development of eye-movement desensitization and reprocessing (EMDR) and acupuncture, and to some extent what is continuing to happen. Both were (and sometimes are) seen as having inexplicable mechanisms of action

http://dx.doi.org/10.1037/0000186-009
Alternative Therapies for PTSD: The Science of Mind–Body Treatments, by R. W. Motta

and thus are placed in the same categories as pseudoscience, voodoo, tea leaf reading, and astrology. Although both still struggle for acceptance within the scientific community, acupuncture has been used by millions and is considered as a viable means of treating many disorders. The U.S. Department of Veterans Affairs accepts EMDR as a valid form of treatment for posttraumatic stress disorder (PTSD; U.S. Department of Veterans Affairs & U.S. Department of Defense, 2017), and EMDR also is accepted by the American Psychological Association (APA) as an empirically supported treatment (EST; APA Presidential Task Force on Evidence-Based Practice, 2006), but many clinicians and researchers continue to see it as a questionable approach. Those adhering to ostensibly orthodox treatment methods are pillorying EFT, one of the newer "kids on the block."

Let's take a look at what this contention might look like. Proponents, opponents, and pragmatists might engage in the following discussion:

PROPONENTS: We have this method of treating psychological and physical disorders based on tapping of meridian end points. It is called EFT. It has been proven in well-controlled studies to be highly effective for alleviating pain and emotional disorders, including PTSD.

OPPONENTS: Your methods are nothing more than pseudoscience and are based on unverifiable meridians, qi, and flawed studies. All of this is mysticism.

PROPONENTS: We use randomly controlled trials and meta-analyses, and we have established a fairly consistent body of positive findings for EFT.

OPPONENTS: The studies and meta-analyses you cite are worthless. A meta-analysis of flawed studies leads to false conclusions.

PROPONENTS: Virtually no studies exist that don't have faults, so using this argument to attack the validity of EFT is disingenuous. Even studies of well-accepted methods, such as cognitive behavior therapy (CBT), have been found to have numerous flaws. One needs to look at the body of supportive EFT evidence, not single studies. This body of evidence supports the efficacy of EFT. In addition, we assert that we meet the criteria set by APA for being an EST.

OPPONENTS: You can't compare EFT to CBT. CBT is based on well-established learning theory and is officially recognized as an EST. EFT is based on unsubstantiated meridians and some unverifiable and mystical body force and the balancing of this supposed force.

PRAGMATISTS: If "unscientific" treatments like EMDR, acupuncture, and EFT work for me, I will use them. I have no problem using a tapping technique for my problems because it helps me. After all, I get great comfort and peace from attending religious services, and yet there is no scientific basis for religion. I can't be bothered by your scientific–unscientific squabbles.

BRIEF HISTORY OF EMOTIONAL FREEDOM TECHNIQUES

EFT began as thought field therapy (TFT) and was developed by psychologist Roger Callahan in 1980 (Callahan & Callahan, 2000). TFT was also known as meridian energy tapping, Callahan techniques, energy therapy, and other terms. Callahan (1997) noticed that by tapping on meridian points on the body, people began to feel better. This has a familiar ring and sounds like the work of Francine Shapiro (2001), who noted that getting people to make saccadic eye movements while thinking about traumatic experiences had a beneficial effect, and from this observation, EMDR evolved. Callahan had a client, Mary, who had a severe water phobia. He found that having her tap below the eye alleviated her fear. Thirty years later, Mary continued to be free of her water fears (Callahan, 1997). Callahan also found that by having people tap various meridian points, many of their psychological and emotional problems were relieved. After his death, Callahan's wife, Joanne Callahan, carried on his work and produced books on energy EFT, positive EFT, and an EFT master course.

In 2016, TFT was listed as an evidence-based treatment by the Substance Abuse and Mental Health Services Administration, an agency of the U.S. Department of Health and Human Services. That agency also found that TFT was effective in treating trauma and stress-related disorders and symptoms, and was helpful in the area of enhancing personal resilience/self-concept (National Psychologist Staff, 2016). Around 2014, Gary Craig, a Stanford University-trained engineer and former student of Callahan, started the popularization of EFT by standardizing the meridian end point tapping sequence for countless problems. Rather than matching a tapping sequence to a specific problem, he developed a general tapping sequence that one could teach and use more easily. In addition, Silvia Hartmann and Chrissie Hardisty founded the Association for Meridian Therapies; the name changed to The Guild of Energists in 2016 ("Developmental History of Energy Tapping Techniques," 2014).

Also, in 2016, a group of American psychologists established the Association for Comprehensive Energy Psychology, and Hartmann wrote the "Meridian Energy Therapy Practitioner" EFT training procedure, which enabled tens of thousands of practitioners to become certified and to subsequently apply for practice insurance ("Developmental History of Energy Tapping Techniques," 2014). Hartmann (2003) also published *Adventures in EFT: Your Essential Guide to Emotional Freedom*, now in its 6th edition. In 2005, Dawson Church began *clinical EFT*, his own version of tapping that was reportedly approved for continuing education credits for psychologists, social workers, and medical practitioners (Church, 2013). Church and David Feinstein (2013) began a series of studies that reportedly culminated in their position that the EFT method met, and in some cases exceeded, the criteria set by the Society of Clinical Psychology (Division 12) of APA (APA Presidential Task Force on Evidence-Based Practice, 2006) as an empirically validated treatment. A plethora of techniques that are variants of EFT go by names that include optimal EFT, classic EFT, clinical EFT, trauma buster technique, simple energy techniques, and matrix reimprinting. It is likely that this wide variety of methods centering around a basic process of tapping on meridians or meridian end points has had both a positive and negative impact. The positive side of things is that the variety has helped spread use of the method. The negative side is that one gets the impression of a cultist slant, which detracts from scientific respectability.

EMOTIONAL FREEDOM TECHNIQUES TREATMENT PROCESS

Before describing relevant research and the specifics of how tapping is done, one needs to first understand that EFT proponents take the position that all negative emotions begin with a disruption of the body energy flow. For this reason, emotional issues, such as depression, anxiety, trauma, and anger, all have a basis in bodily energy disruption. And, because many physical problems are exacerbated by or have their origins in emotional distress, EFT often relieves them, too. EFT encompasses four steps.

Step 1: Identify the Problem

First, the trauma sufferer or client identifies a target problem. Problems may be: "My sore hand," "My horrific experience of having to fire at someone in Iraq," "My mother humiliated me in front of my friends when I was 10."

Step 2: Rate the Intensity of the Problem

On a Subjective Units of Distress Scale (Wolpe & Lazarus, 1966), the client attempts to give an intensity rating to the problem they are dealing with. This rating is most often on a scale from 1 (*none or almost none*) to 10 (*maximum or most intense*). If a problem starts as a 10 and diminishes to a 5 with repeated tapping, then 50% improvement has occurred. The point is an attempt is made to provide a somewhat objective rating to the level of distress and its improvement. So, for an emotional issue, one would replay the situation to which they are reacting and then provide a rating. For a physical issue, such as pain, one tries to rate it from no pain, a 1, to intense pain, a 10. If the issue happens to involve dissatisfaction with one's performance at a task or sport, again a low rating would indicate being extremely dissatisfied with one's performance, and a high rating, being satisfied with one's performance.

Step 3: Begin the Setup Phase

This step is referred to as the *setup* and is used in the beginning of each tapping session. The purpose of the setup is to acknowledge rather than deny the existence of a specific personal problem and to follow that acknowledgment with a clear statement of self-acceptance. Two elements compose the setup phase:

- Acknowledging the problem: "Even though I _____ (*fill in the blank*)." The statement of the problem would go in the blank. For example, "I regret having made an incorrect business decision," "I am annoyed that my neck is hurting," "I participated in that dumb escapade," or any other problem or difficulty.

- Accepting yourself despite the problem: For example, "I deeply and completely accept myself" (Ortner, 2013, p. 18).

- So, statements might look like the following:
  - "Even though I have a fear of driving, I deeply and completely accept myself."
  - "Even though I have this knee pain, I deeply and completely accept myself."
  - "Even though I failed my licensing exam, I deeply and completely accept myself."
  - "Even though I was abused as a child, I deeply and completely accept myself."

It is important that the setup statement be an issue relevant to the client and not to someone else. So, it is inadvisable to use a statement like, "Even though my wife has a drinking problem, I deeply and completely accept myself." It would be more desirable to have a setup statement like, "Even though I spend my days obsessing about my wife's drinking, I deeply and completely accept myself." The identified problem must be one's own, and not another person's, difficulties.

The second part of this statement is important in that many forms of emotional and physical problems involve a form of self-negation or denigration that the client must overcome to move forward. It is important that we accept ourselves as fallible human beings who are prone to mistakes, misjudgments, errors, and so on, including the mistake of negatively judging ourselves. If after acknowledging the problem, self-acceptance just seems too difficult to handle, particularly in early phases, it may be temporarily omitted. Also, note that the language identifies a negative experience that is causing the "energy flow" problem. Many self-help approaches emphasize the positive, but adherents to EFT view doing so as covering up rather than directly addressing one's problems. So, in EFT, one acknowledges that a problem of some kind exists, but there is a self-acceptance and no minimization or denial of a problem.

To some extent, this acknowledgment of the problem might be seen as an exposure component, and it is. We are reexposing ourselves to a problem. "When you tap while recalling and upsetting scene from your childhood, you are doing a modified version of exposure therapy. The exposure happens when you think about the upsetting scene. Tapping often retrains the limbic system rapidly" (Ortner, 2013, p. 8). Having said this, exposure to traumatic experiences has been identified as one of the major reasons why people avoid therapies for PTSD. Confronting traumatic experiences again causes extreme levels of anxiety. So why are we including a method of treating PTSD that involves exposure in EFT? The reason is that, unlike traditional approaches, such as CBT, the traumatized individual does not have to engage in a detailed immersion of the prior trauma as is done in the more typical exposure-based therapies. Traditional therapies often require a detailed revisiting of the trauma, including the sights, sounds, smells, and extreme emotions associated with the trauma, and by repeating this process, the client becomes desensitized to these difficult-to-tolerate elements. EFT, and to some extent EMDR, though, do not proceed in this manner. Neither EFT nor EMDR involve such detailed recalling of traumatic experiences, and, in this way, are said to evoke less of an avoidance response. Because of the lack of detail and reimmersion into formerly traumatic events, EFT may be said to sidestep the negative aspects of traditional exposure procedures.

Step 4: Start the Tapping Process

Although the literature may vary on the specific sequence of tapping, one can begin with the karate chop (see Figure 8.1a). To do the karate chop, one uses the index and middle finger of one hand while tapping the fleshy part of the other hand approximately five to seven times. So, the karate chop involves tapping while saying, "Even though I was once arrested, I deeply and completely accept myself," while tapping five to seven times. This process is repeated about three times but can be done more than that if the individual is highly distressed. One then goes through the various tapping points (see Figure 8.1b) while using a *reminder phrase*, a brief restatement. So, while tapping the top of the head five to seven times, one might say, "My arrest" or "My abuse" or "My shoulder pain" or "My overeating."

The client repeats this reminder phrase as they progress through the various body parts identified in Figure 8.1b:

- top of the head;

- beginning of the eyebrow, that is, the point where either eyebrow begins;

FIGURE 8.1. The Tapping Process Showing Points for the Karate Chop (a) and From the Waist Up (b)

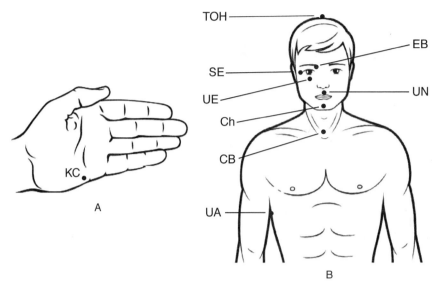

CB = beginning of the collarbone; Ch = chin; EB = beginning of the eyebrow; KC = karate chop; SE = side of the eye; TOH = top of the head; UA = under the arm; UE = under the eye; UN = under the nose.

- side of the eye, where one taps the bony structure—the orbit—at the outside of either eye;

- under the eye, where tapping occurs again on the bony structure just below the eye;

- under the nose, where one taps between the bottom of the nose and the upper lip;

- chin, where tapping occurs between the lower lip and the tip of the chin;

- beginning of the collarbone, where one first locates the notch at the center of the collarbone and then taps at the beginning of the collarbone; and

- under the arm; the point for men is under the armpit from a line drawn across from the nipple; for women, it is the point where the bra strap goes over the upper ribcage.

A number of videos, such as those on YouTube, can provide instruction on the tapping process. Instructional resources are also provided in the Appendix to this book.

At this point, the client reassesses the level of distress they presented in Step 2: They determine a rating of discomfort on the 1-to-10 Subjective Units of Distress Scale (Wolpe & Lazarus, 1966). If there is no change or insufficient change, then they repeat the whole process, going from the top of the head to under the arm while tapping and stating the reminder phrase. The goal is to move to a level of 1 or 2.

Review of the Emotional Freedom Techniques Process

The material that follows is a guide. These are the locations of the various body tapping points used in EFT:

- nine primary tapping points: karate chop, top of the head, beginning of the eyebrow, side of the eye, under the eye, under the nose, chin, beginning of the collarbone, under the arm;

- setup phrase used with the karate chop;

- reminder phrase used with the remainder of the tapping points;

- measurement of the intensity on the 1-to-10 Subjective Units of Distress Scale (Wolpe & Lazarus, 1966) just before the karate chop and after under the arm; and

- continuation of tapping through the nine points until distress approaches 1 on the scale.

Given that meridians are reportedly arranged symmetrically on both sides of the body, one can, for example, tap on the beginning of the eyebrow of either eye. It does not matter which hand the client uses. If one wishes to tap both sides, that is also acceptable because the issue is to free up energy transmission. One taps with two or more fingertips to assure that the specific point is stimulated. Some people may have difficulty finding the collarbone point. It is acceptable to use a closed fist and tap the center depression between the collarbones to assure that collarbone stimulation takes place. Tapping can be done anywhere in the range of 3 to 7 times, except during the setup phase in which one engages in continuous tapping while repeating the setup statement. Like many of the alternative methods presented in this book, advanced levels of training are available for those interested in practicing EFT or treating others with this method. The interested reader can find additional resources in the literature, such as Ortner's (2013, 2015) texts and the documentary "The Tapping Solution" (2008).

CASE EXAMPLE: TREATING THE TRAUMA OF CHILD LOSS WITH EMOTIONAL FREEDOM TECHNIQUES

Nick and Tammy have lived through one of the most painful experiences that parents can endure: the loss of a child. They had a boy and two girls, and had formed a close-knit, loving family. Their family did not reach whatever the mythical ideal might be but rather encountered typical conflicts and stresses, such as dealing with teens who pressed for autonomy and adjusting to their new home in Colorado, having recently moved from New York. Their son, Tom, age 19, grew up to be a shy, socially awkward, and yet loving young man who ran into conflict with his dad because of Tom's pressing for more independence and freedom. Eventually, Nick relented, and Tom got his own apartment, where he often engaged in partying and drinking with several of his close friends. One evening, coming back from a camping trip and maybe still a bit under the influence, he was driving at his usual breakneck pace. He failed to negotiate a tight mountain curve, and his car hit an embankment and flipped over, throwing Tom to the pavement. The EMT who arrived on the scene did not feel optimistic about Tom's chances of survival. He was nonresponsive and bleeding profusely from a head injury.

Doctors and medical staff in the intensive care unit worked long into the night, but they were unable to overcome a decisive and painful reality. Tom was not showing the signs of a functioning brain. He was brain dead. Recovery was impossible. Nick and Tammy had spent the evening in the hospital praying, hoping, pacing, holding each other, and sobbing with fear. When the neurosurgeon walked into the waiting area and delivered the terrible news, Nick and Tammy's world collapsed. Stunned disbelief followed along with a hollow sense of dread that they would have to continue living without their son. Tom's body was kept alive by machines for 3 days in a desperate and unlikely hope for recovery. They made the painful decision to disconnect Tom when it became apparent that he would not recover. Having to outlive your children is simply a living hell. The dread and emptiness of facing each day without one's child or children is unimaginably painful, and the suffering lessens at a grindingly slow pace over time.

Tom's parents managed the endless days of pain differently. Tammy stayed close to her friends and was constantly socially engaged. This activity and her involvement in her daughters' lives helped distract her, but she carried a constant sadness with her. Nick did less well and sought to deaden his pain with long, isolated walks; drinking; smoking marijuana; and eating binges. However, he did participate in bereavement groups. He gained a considerable amount of weight, and developed gout and blood pressure and blood sugar problems. Headaches, fatigue, and sleepless followed. His distraction caused a failure of his realty business, and he entertained secret thoughts of how to make his suicide look like an accident. Jumping in front of a passing car was one of his preferred suicidal strategies. His pain seemed unabated even with the passage of 10 years. He pushed through life, but, by his own admission, had little will to live. Being out of work did not help matters. The distraction of work demands would have allowed him to spend a little less time dwelling on the negatives of his existence.

While looking to purchase an electrical stimulation device to help with his gout, he obtained the name of a German salesperson living in Canada. As it happened, the salesperson, Christina, had been trained in EFT. She advised Nick that this procedure might be effective in helping him release his pain. Nick proceeded to engage in tapping sessions over the phone with Christina's guidance. During their first of three sessions, Nick sobbed uncontrollably while going through the tapping sequence. By the fourth session, the sobbing had stopped, and in Nick's words, the tapping helped him "emotionally release" and "rid myself of years of pent-up pain." Although the tapping involved a setup statement like "Although I deeply grieve the loss of my son . . .," Nick vehemently asserts that it was not this cognitive restatement that helped him. Nick identifies the release of the dammed emotion that helped him move forward.

Nick's recovery has been slow, but what started to happen is that he began to replace unhealthy habits with healthy ones. He radically reduced his drinking and drug use, and he oriented himself toward a plant-based, nutritious diet. He began regular sessions of meditation with his wife, Tammy. Their relationship, characterized by distance and isolation after their son's death, became closer and more intimate. It appeared that the emotional release, the undamming of the blocked pain, served as a catalyst for movement in a healthy direction. Nick and Tammy will never forget the pain of losing their son, but that pain is now more manageable, and they are able to move on with their lives.

One of the issues that began to stand out in my discussions with Nick is that what took place in his EFT sessions was entirely focused on the release of blocked emotions and not a focal reorienting of cognitions and behaviors. Consider for a moment CBT. As the term *cognitive behavior therapy* implies, the focus is directly on how one thinks and on the replacement of irrational thoughts with rational ones. One also tries to identify flaws in their thinking, such as personalizing everything, thinking in black-and-white terms, and over-generalizing. In CBT, one makes an attempt to realize that all is not personal; that things are not bad or good but that gradations exist; and that one should not generalize a failure at a task, for example, to seeing themselves as a failure overall. Similarly, CBT emphasizes engaging in adaptive behaviors. These behavioral adaptations might be such things as socializing more, behaving more assertively, or confronting uncomfortable challenges. EFT has an entirely different focus.

From the EFT perspective, negative life events can cause a blockage of emotion and bodily energies. This energy is the qi of Eastern perspectives. The tapping on the various meridian endpoints unblocks the emotions and facilitates energy transfer. What follows is a growth in emotional and physical well-being. This perspective is like that what occurs when a person has a physical wound: The body has a natural tendency toward health. Given the right conditions, the wound heals automatically. Similarly, in EFT, when one unblocks the pent-up energy and emotion, healing takes place. It is certainly understandable that Western-trained clinicians and researchers have difficulty with this kind of explanation. Little hard data verify qi, meridians, or this mysterious flow of energy. And yet the empirical research does show that EFT provides measurable healthy outcomes for those suffering from trauma and pain of various kinds.

EMDR, like EFT, goes about dealing with trauma in different ways than does CBT. EMDR methods put a good deal of emphasis on the human body and mind's tendency to self-heal, and both EMDR and EFT assert that once this healing takes place, there is little relapse. The mind and body, or bodymind, to use Candace Pert's (1999) term—the unity of these hypothesized separate entities—will heal once the energies can be unblocked, or, in EMDR's terms, once the information processing parts of the brain can be unblocked. CBT takes the view that emotional pain is results from cognitive misrepresentations or distortions. The goal of therapy is then to create healthier, more adaptive cognitions and also engage in healthy adaptive behaviors. EFT seems to place a greater emphasis on automated mind–body processes, whereas CBT stresses intentional and willful efforts to change how one goes about their life. CBT appears to fit in with the Western view of self-determination, whereas EFT emphasizes energy blockages and a healing process that is perhaps built-in, automatic, and somewhat beyond one's will. These are very different orientations. For Nick, EFT as an alternative to traditional CBT was the way home. For many others, CBT may be the right road. There seems to be no one right path. And alternative approaches are available, which is the focus of this volume. It is important for clinicians and especially for researchers to be open to novel approaches if the data support these new methods. Many traditionalists will write off EFT as palmistry, but the ever-accumulating data make that an increasingly difficult position to maintain. Increasing numbers of therapists are beginning to use and accept EFT (Gaudiano, Brown, & Miller, 2012).

SCIENTIFIC STUDIES OF TREATMENTS FOR PTSD, INCLUDING NONTRADITIONAL INTERVENTIONS

As with the other alternative therapeutic approaches previously covered, no one generally agrees on the mechanism of action for EFT. Meridians, qi, energy flow, and energy blockages are the explanatory approaches. Similarly, EMDR uses an information-processing model whereby areas of the brain, such as the prefrontal cortex, are reactivated, and lower centers, like the amygdala, are muted. Exercise, yoga, and meditation may rely on various body–mind unifications to explain their effects, but these explanations are difficult to verify. Acupuncture and EFT appear to have similar explanatory constructs, but it is unclear that these constructs are difficult to verify. One might reasonably ask, "Where's the proof?" "Where is the science in all of this?" Again, the pragmatist might not care, but those who have been professionally trained often wish to know about the bases of change or whether there is any real change beyond illusion, hope, belief, or placebo. The material in this section is oriented toward a deeper investigation of the science behind EFT, even if the explanatory mechanisms remain unclear.

CBT is considered to be the treatment of choice by many in the psychotherapy field. However, as indicated in Chapter 1, many find the treatment difficult to tolerate because it often entails an immersion into one's prior traumatic experiences, and the difficulty in carrying this out can frequently eventuate in fleeing therapy. Most people who start treatment for psychological difficulties quit for a variety of reasons. The majority of those who begin treatment for PTSD quit because of the treatment itself. Confronting the trauma experiences again is simply too difficult to tolerate.

Meta-Analysis of Emotional Freedom Techniques for PTSD

Recall that meta-analysis combines the results of many studies and, as such, avoids the common critique that every study has its flaws. By combining data from many studies, one obtains an overall, and generally less biased, view of findings. A meta-analysis of EFT for PTSD of veterans from wars in Iraq and Afghanistan and other nonwar PTSD sufferers was conducted by Sebastian and Nelms (2017). These authors indicated that EFT uses exposure and cognitive reprocessing. The exposure component involves a restatement of the traumatic experience, although not an in-depth one. For example, a setup statement in EFT might be, "Although I fired my weapon at insurgents in Iraq, I deeply and completely accept myself." The cognitive reprocessing part may be the acceptance segment of the setup. Rather than view oneself in a negative self-rejecting light, the trauma victim makes a statement of self-acceptance. "Then the client taps, massages, or holds a set of acupoints" (Sebastian & Nelms, 2017, p. 17), and provides a Subjective Units of Distress Scale (Wolpe & Lazarus, 1966) rating of 1 to 10. The client completes rounds of EFT as just described until the veteran is able to bring forward the memory of what happened with little to no subjective distress.

In their meta-analysis, Sebastian and Nelms (2017) sought to include only studies that met evidence-based criteria set by the Society of Clinical Psychology (Division 12) of APA (APA Presidential Task Force on Evidence-Based Practice, 2006). These criteria involve such procedures as random assignment to conditions, adequate sample size to detect differences between groups, and reliable and valid assessment tools. The authors identified seven randomized controlled trials that met the APA criteria. They found a large treatment effect (2.96) for studies that compared EFT with usual care or wait-list. No treatment effect differences were found in studies comparing EFT with other evidence-based therapies, such as EMDR and CBT. Sebastian and Nelms concluded that

> the analysis of existing studies showed that a series of 4–10 EFT sessions is an efficacious treatment for PTSD with a variety of populations. The studies examined reported no adverse effects from EFT interventions and showed that it can be used both on a self-help basis and as a primary evidence-based treatment for PTSD. (p. 16)

It is important to consider the implications of the concluding statement by Sebastian and Nelms (2017). First, the fact that only four to 10 sessions of EFT were required to bring about efficacious treatment of PTSD is surprising. It is not unusual for PTSD to last for a lifetime and for treatment to go on for many years. I will never forget an 87-year-old veteran of World War II saying to me, "Doc, what am I going to do about this damn PTSD?" He had been suffering for most of his life. If there are validated treatments for PTSD that can be concluded in 10 sessions or fewer, this is a remarkable achievement. And yet, much of the scientific and clinical community sees EFT as voodoo. That the method is fairly easily taught and can be used as a "self-help" technique is also profound. What this means is that those who do not have access to psychotherapy services or resources to support ongoing psychological intervention, medical intervention, or both, have a way of dealing with the torment of PTSD.

EFT has been found to be comparable and, in some cases, more effective than "gold standard" treatment, such as CBT. It also has been found to be equally as effective as EMDR, a treatment that has also struggled with acceptability because of its unorthodox methodology and explanatory constructs (Gaesser & Karan, 2017). The EMDR and CBT approaches require trained clinicians. EFT does not make this demand and can be engaged in on a self-care basis. Traditionalists clearly do not want to hear such things. It is threatening. I vividly recall the outrage that some expressed when a doctoral candidate and I presented data at a formal psychology convention showing that aerobic exercise was equally effective as CBT in reducing depression. Findings that favorably compare self-help methods, such as exercise, yoga, and meditation, with traditional interventions for psychological disorders simply do not sit well with many professionals.

"Hard Science" Behind Emotional Freedom Techniques

Growing evidence from "hard science" investigations of the impact of EFT includes, for example, studies involving functional magnetic resonance imaging procedures that have shown that stimulating acupoints downgrades limbic system activity, primarily the amygdala (Dhond, Kettner, & Napadow, 2007). Other studies (e.g., Fox, 2013) have shown that acupoint stimulation of the type seen in both EFT and acupuncture releases serotonin in the amygdala and prefrontal cortex, resulting in a rapid reduction in hyperarousal. In addition, stimulation of acupoints leads to the release of serotonin, opioids, serotonin, and gamma-aminobutyric acid; the result is a slowing down of the fight–flight–freeze response and heart rate, as well as a reduction in pain and anxiety (Sebastian & Nelms, 2017; Varvogli & Darviri, 2011).

In a well-controlled and blinded study, Church, Yount, and Brooks (2012) tested saliva to measure cortisol levels and compared EFT with a no-treatment group and a supportive interview. They found that cortisol decreased equally (14%) for both the no-treatment group and the supportive intervention but 24% after a single 1-hour session in the EFT group (Sebastian & Nelms, 2017).

Using electroencephalography, studies have mapped brain waves and shown that electroencephalography frequencies associated with relaxation (theta waves) are associated with EFT tapping (Lembrou, Pratt, & Chevalier, 2003). One study (Swingle, Pulos, & Swingle, 2003) that examined car accident survivors at risk for PTSD found that brain frequencies linked with fear have been reduced after EFT (Sebastian & Nelms, 2017).

Opponents of Emotional Freedom Techniques

It is rare, if not unheard of, for a new treatment to present itself without vigorous opposition from the scientific community. Institutions, particularly universities that are oriented toward empirically sound research methods, are highly conservative and resistant to change. They have a natural opposition to new and unorthodox methods. Such was, and to some is, the case with EMDR, which used the unusual procedure of alternating visual, kinesthetic, or auditory stimulation. EFT is no exception. EFT has been referred to as a threat to the science of psychology and psychiatry. Bakker (2013) suggested that the evidence for energy psychology studies such as EFT is a "swamp" and has advocated a halt to any research on these methods because they are unlikely to be productive. Others find the growing popularity of methods such as EFT to be nothing short of alarming and a threat to both science and reason. They contend that the fast-growing acceptance by the clinical community of such methods as EFT is because the therapists who use these methods are far more gullible and less rigorous in their treatment choice decisions than those who are scientifically oriented. Others cite the high failure rate of new therapies and this, along with institutional inertia, has been shown to delay the adoption of new approaches to clinical practice by an average of 17 years (Church, Feinstein, Palmer-Hoffman, Stein, & Tranguch, 2014). The process of adaptation to change often occurs at a glacial pace. Acupuncture, despite its wide usage across the globe, is still seen as mystical and unscientific by many. EMDR, an empirically validated treatment by APA (APA Presidential Task Force on Evidence-Based Practice, 2006) is viewed as pseudoscience by academics who have not taken the time to acquaint themselves with its methods but rather have reflexively responded with opposition. That is where EFT currently is. It is seen as existing in a pseudoscience swamp despite the existence of quite a large number of well-controlled studies attesting to its efficacy, utility, and accessibility. All of this makes one wonder about the true objectivity of "science," but that is another matter.

EMPIRICAL RESEARCH OF ACTIVE INGREDIENTS IN EMOTIONAL FREEDOM TECHNIQUES

A number of studies show that EFT produces improvements in anxiety, depression, phobias, and PTSD. It has also produced improvements in physical conditions, such as fibromyalgia, psoriasis, tension headaches, pain, traumatic brain injury, and seizure disorders (e.g., Bougea et al., 2013). A question remains: Is acupressure an essential ingredient in EFT, or do the effects of acupressure result from its cognitive- and exposure-based elements or factors that all therapies have in common, such as an expectation of positive outcomes (i.e., placebo effects) or sympathetic attention (Church & Nelms, 2016)?

To address the "active ingredient" question, a study was conducted involving limited range of motion in the shoulder, also called "frozen shoulder." Church and Nelms (2016) assigned 37 participants randomly to one of three conditions. Condition 1 was EFT. Condition 2 was EFT without the tapping but substituting diaphragmatic breathing for tapping. The point of having this condition was to determine if the tapping itself did anything over and above such EFT procedures as setup statements. This process of isolating therapeutic elements to determine their efficacy, or lack thereof, is called a *dismantling procedure*. Condition 3 was a wait-list control that is used to see if any form of treatment is better than no treatment.

Multiple measures of pain, motion, and a variety of psychological symptoms were obtained in a pre–posttest format, and the data were analyzed in a blind fashion (i.e., data analysts were not informed of the condition from which the data were obtained; Church & Nelms, 2016). Results showed that no statistically significant improvements were shown in the wait-list condition. Participants in the EFT group (Group 1) and diaphragmatic breathing substitution group (Group 2) demonstrated statistically significant improvements in pain and psychological symptoms. Follow-up revealed that the EFT and diaphragmatic breathing substitution groups had continued gains for pain—and EFT was superior to the second group; however, only the EFT group had continued gains for psychological symptoms. Church and Nelms (2016) found statistically large EFT treatment effects for pain, depression, and anxiety. For most measures in the groups, range of motion changes were not statistically significant. The study authors concluded,

> EFT can reduce pain in a brief treatment time frame, and produces durable improvements in psychological conditions such as anxiety and depression. It strengthens the case for clinical EFT as an evidence-based practice and shows that its acupoint tapping component is an active ingredient in the manualized protocol. (p. 46)

Church and Nelms (2016) convincingly demonstrated that tapping was an active and important ingredient in EFT. They also demonstrated that reductions in psychological symptoms, anxiety, and depression, the critical components of PTSD, were maintained over a 30-day period. The treatment changes were both statistically significant and demonstrated large effect sizes (approximately 1.0, or twice as large as that typically judged as clinically effective). A further and equally impressive finding of this study is that all of these beneficial changes took place within a single 30-minute session. Standard psychological treatments for anxiety and depression can take months or even years of weekly sessions. To obtain significant reductions that are maintained over time in one 30-minute session is, if valid, most impressive. One might argue that a 30-day follow-up is insufficient, and yet this is a standard used in many evaluations of traditional treatments.

Further Empirical Research on Emotional Freedom Techniques With PTSD

The Church and Nelms (2016) study noted that EFT was highly effective in reducing the PTSD symptoms of anxiety, depression, and a number of other distressing symptoms despite its limited efficacy improving range of motion of those with frozen shoulder syndrome. In another study, EFT demonstrated a direct impact on PTSD among war veterans (Church et al., 2013). Setup statements in that study were of the following nature: "Even though I had to shoot insurgents firing at us, I deeply and completely accept myself." And a reminder statement while going through the tapping might be, "Shooting at insurgents."

Fifteen providers performed EFT; each coached between one and 12 veterans, and the mean was four veterans (Church et al., 2013). Of interest is that although the coaches were trained in EFT, they were not all doctoral-level providers. Half had master's degrees, two had bachelor's degrees, two had associate's degrees, and one had no degree but had some college background. Three practitioners were registered nurses. One can only imagine the possible resistance from doctoral-level or other professionally trained providers that this assortment of ranges of training might evoke. One does not have to be professionally trained to use EFT treatment. The benefit is that EFT can be made widely available. The downside is that the lack of required professional training to do EFT treatment may detract from the perceived validity of the procedure.

In the Church et al. (2013) study, 30 veterans received EFT and were compared with 29 who received standard care and were standard of care wait-list controls, and random assignment was used. The study required all participants to be under the care of a clinician from the Department of Veterans Affairs or other licensed health care facility. The EFT coaching intervention was delivered as a complementary and supportive supplement to the standard of care. All participants were diagnosed with PTSD using standardized valid and reliable measures. The EFT intervention was six hour-long coaching sessions. The results following blind data analysis showed that the EFT group had significantly reduced psychological distress and PTSD symptom levels. In addition, 90% of the EFT group no longer met clinical criteria for PTSD compared with 4% of the standard of care wait-list group. After the researchers had obtained these data, they then provided participants in the standard of care wait-list group with EFT, and, after three sessions, 60% no longer showed PTSD symptoms. This figure increased to 86% after six sessions. The authors state that the results were "consistent with that of other published reports showing EFT's efficacy in treating PTSD and comorbid symptoms and its long-term effects" (Church et al., 2013, p. 153).

That dramatic results were noted after six sessions of treatment is of no small consequence. Actually, the study noted improvements after three sessions (Church et al., 2013). The dropout rate was low compared with that typically seen in Department of Veterans Affairs treatments of PTSD. The low dropout rate might be the result of the perception of a peer-to-peer rather than a professional-to-peer therapeutic arrangement. Regardless of the reasons, what the Church et al. (2013) study demonstrates is a high level of treatment acceptability from those being treated. Although this study, like most other psychological studies, can be critiqued on a whole range of methodological grounds, it does add to the growing body of evidence showing that EFT can be effective in treating PTSD. The results of the study indicate that a six-session intervention of EFT provided essentially by life coaches can be a useful intervention for veterans. Ninety percent who were formerly diagnosed with PTSD no longer met the criteria for this disorder after six sessions. The study authors noted that further research is needed to determine the comparable effectiveness of group versus individual EFT intervention and the degree to which professional training has an impact on the efficacy of EFT.

Emotional Freedom Techniques With School-Age Children

More than 50 million school-age children attend pre-K to high school in the United States, and more than 5 million experience troubling anxiety levels (Costello, Mustillo, Erkanli, Keeler, & Angold, 2003). About 2.5 million refuse to go to school, participate in school activities, or both because of the disabling effects of anxiety (Gaesser & Karan, 2017). In a randomized controlled study, Gaesser and Karan (2017) randomly assigned 62 high-ability children ranging in age from 10 to 18 years old to an EFT condition, a CBT condition adapted for children, or a wait-list control. All children selected for the study were given a standardized anxiety measure, the Revised Children's Manifest Anxiety Scale (Reynolds & Richmond, 1985) and were selected if they scored in the moderate-to-high level of anxiety at the start of the study. Children received three individual sessions of EFT or CBT over a 5-month period; the wait-list control did not receive any intervention but simply completed the anxiety measure. Those who were blind as to the study conditions analyzed data. The results showed that EFT participants showed significantly reduced anxiety levels compared with the wait-list control, and with a moderate-to-large effect size. CBT participants showed reductions in anxiety but did not significantly differ from the EFT or control condition.

Results of the Gaesser and Karan (2017) study demonstrate that EFT can be an effective treatment of childhood and adolescent anxiety, and the findings support similar studies showing that EFT is an evidence-based intervention for adolescent anxiety and test anxiety, and also reduces the intensity of traumatic memories in abused adolescents (Church, Piña, Reategui, & Brooks, 2012). According to Gaesser and Karan, one of the reasons that EFT was shown to be effective is that it incorporates a somatic component. The body component in this study was the stimulation of acupoints. The literature increasingly shows that adding a somatic component to therapy is becoming increasingly popular. When acupoint stimulation is added to standard exposure therapy, the extinction of fear memories is accelerated (Harper, 2012). Furthermore, biophysiological markers of stress reduction following EFT have included normalization of brain wave patterns and hormonal changes.

The view of the importance of adding a somatic component to therapy is certainly in accord with studies of EMDR in which attention is paid to how the body is responding to traumatic memories. It also is in line with the earlier case example of Nick and Tammy, who lost their son in an automobile accident. According to Nick, the therapeutic element that helped him move forward was the emotional release following from the body tapping of meridian end points done using EFT. Whether one is a proponent or opponent of energy therapies, such as EFT, there does seem to be something important to be said about the therapeutic value of incorporating the body in the treatment of trauma. Body components are seldom addressed in traditional CBT other than in reference to diaphragmatic breathing and relaxation. EFT emphasizes the somatic component through tapping, and according to van der Kolk (2014), the body does keep score, at least as far as trauma is concerned. Gaesser and Karan (2017) suggested that a minimally intrusive procedure like EFT might effectively address a major impediment to school functioning involving millions of children and without causing significant interruption of the normal school day:

> Results of this study are consistent with findings from previous research and a meta-analysis showing the EFT is an efficacious, evidence-based treatment for adolescent anxiety. Additionally, the results indicate that EFT can be effectively used in school settings to significantly reduce adolescent anxiety with a few sessions. (p. 106)

Now, as compelling as the Gaesser and Karan (2017) study of the use of EFT with children and adolescents may be, it is possible for EFT opponents to critique it on a number of grounds: The sample size was relatively small and may not be representative of children overall. The study was conducted with high-ability children who might react differently to EFT and CBT than average to lower ability youngsters. The study authors used only one anxiety measure, and although it was reliable and valid, it is often recommended that multiple measures be used, including physiological measures, such as cortisol or galvanic skin response. The study involved only three sessions, and usually CBT is administered in a larger number of sessions, so the Gaesser and Karan study might not accurately represent the reputed "gold standard" effects of CBT. That study, like all others, has its strengths and weaknesses. However, as stated earlier, one should never judge an intervention based on a single study. One must examine a body of research conducted with different samples and using different methods for a myriad of problems. Meta-analyses should be conducted to evaluate the accumulated body of evidence. When these recommendations are followed, the overall thrust of findings appears to support the utility of EFT as an intervention for trauma and trauma-related disorders.

STRENGTH OF EMPIRICAL SUPPORT

EFT has received fairly strong empirical support and shows effect sizes comparable with those of CBT and EMDR. Such impressive support may seem surprising to those who find the procedure to be relatively unknown to the majority of clinicians and to those who find no Western-based explanation for EFT's efficacy. EFT, like acupuncture, is based on an explanatory model involving the unblocking of an energy flow. Although there seems little (Western) support for this model, compelling evidence points to the utility of EFT in treating emotional issues, such as PTSD, anxiety, and depression, as well as physical problems related to pain. Hard data show both chemical and physiological changes as a result of EFT. Its proponents report that it meets all criteria set by the APA for ESTs. Its detractors, perhaps unfairly, level the same pseudoscience accusation at EFT that was leveled at EMDR, a treatment now accepted by APA.

SUMMARY

EFT is a recently developed intervention that has demonstrated its utility in managing a variety of disorders. Its newness and its unorthodox methods have served to evoke protests and scoffing among traditionally trained researchers, academics, and, to a lesser extent, clinicians. Given that approximately 30 such "energy therapies" emphasize the stimulation of meridian points and that these meridians are difficult to validate adds fuel to the fire of the opposition to the procedures. A similar opposition was evoked in response to EMDR, despite its being recognized as a respected procedure by many professional organizations, including APA. The reality is that many continue to see EMDR as pseudoscience. Given this resistance, it seems highly likely that opposition to EFT will continue for years to come.

Despite this resistance, it is hard to ignore EFT. Its proponents have gone to considerable lengths using randomly controlled trials, meta-analyses, and both physiological and psychological forms of measurement to demonstrate its utility. The practicing clinician, even the skeptical one, would be well advised to add EFT to their clinical tool kit in treating those clients who may have not responded to other methods. Exposure forms of therapy are often seen as difficult to tolerate. Both CBT and EMDR are somewhat complex and demand a fair amount of training to effectively implement. EFT is a simpler form of intervention that can be administered by those without credentialed professional training. It typically requires few sessions, and initial reports support a resistance to relapse, much like EMDR. The primary goal of clinicians is to help clients. If EFT, or EMDR, or exercise, or yoga, or any of the other interventions covered to this point are going to move the client in the direction of healthy adjustment, then it behooves clinicians to give these interventions serious consideration.

9

MDMA ("Ecstasy") for PTSD

It is reasonable to ask why an illegal street and party drug is being included as one of the alternative treatments for posttraumatic stress disorder (PTSD). The answer is that psychiatrists and clinicians had been using MDMA—3,4-methylenedioxymethamphetamine—which also is called "Adam," "Ecstasy," and "Molly" in the rave and party scene, for years as an aid to psychotherapy, especially in the treatment of psychological trauma. Notably, however, MDMA differs from Ecstasy in that Ecstasy is often adulterated with other drugs, is seldom a pure form of MDMA, and is most often used for nontherapeutic purposes. The use of MDMA as a facilitator for psychotherapy continued until the drug was classified as a Schedule I controlled substance in 1985 under the federal Controlled Substances Act of 1970 of the U.S. Drug Enforcement Administration. Schedule I substances are federally banned.

Another reason for the growing interest in MDMA is that the U.S. Food and Drug Administration (FDA) is now overseeing Phase III clinical trials of MDMA given that initial studies have demonstrated its value as a therapeutic adjunct in treating PTSD. Despite its psychotherapeutic promise, many would consider its use as a treatment of PTSD as a last resort in that MDMA is not easily administered. Treatment involves the use of a banned substance administered over a period of days or weeks by a trained and appropriately certified psychotherapy team, and the treatment must occur with the ready availability of medical oversight. After approximately three, 8-hours sessions using MDMA over a period of weeks, a period of an additional 8 to 16 weeks of nondrug psychotherapy sessions follows. Overall, MDMA treatment can be highly

http://dx.doi.org/10.1037/0000186-010
Alternative Therapies for PTSD: The Science of Mind–Body Treatments, by R. W. Motta

effective even in the most resistant of PTSD cases, but it is a difficult treatment package to put together.

Schedule I of the Controlled Substances Act of 1970 includes substances that the United States currently does not accept as having medical use, those that are not acceptably safe to use under medical supervision, and substances likely to be abused (Robotti, 2019). Examples of substances listed in Schedule I are MDMA, marijuana (cannabis), heroin, lysergic acid diethylamide (LSD), peyote, and methaqualone (Quaalude; Robotti, 2019). The Act categorizes drugs on five levels based on their risk of abuse or harm. It bans high-risk substances having no counterbalancing benefit from medical practice; these substances are Schedule I drugs (Robotti, 2019). The use and abuse of Ecstasy in the club and rave scenes, and the attendant medical problems that over-dosing produced led the federal government to ban MDMA. It was seen as both dangerous and as having no medical value. One can reasonably question the logic for banning some of the drugs mentioned earlier and categorizing them as Schedule I substances. Whether right or wrong, MDMA is, as of this writing, federally banned.

OVERVIEW OF MDMA'S DEVELOPMENT, USAGE, AND EFFECTS

MDMA was initially developed in the laboratory somewhat by accident when the pharmaceutical company Merck was attempting to synthesize a vaso-constrictor and styptic drug of the type that might be used to stop the bleeding from cuts while shaving (Bernschneider-Reif, Oxler, & Freudenmann, 2006). Merck filed a patent application in 1912; Kaiserliches Pantentamt granted it in 1914 ("File: Merck Patent," 1914; Holland, 2001). The finding that MDMA was profoundly psychoactive was entirely serendipitous, but clinicians began to raise questions about whether it could be of psychotherapeutic value. In the 1970s and 1980s, psychiatrists and other clinicians were using the drug—then called "Adam"—as a way of lowering defenses and allowing clients to deal with long-repressed memories (National Institute on Drug Abuse, n.d.). Recall that one of the major problems in treating those who have PTSD is that they vigorously and reflexively avoid painful memories, both consciously and unconsciously. Under the influence of MDMA, at levels lower than used in rave settings, clients became able to view these memories without the anxiety and avoidance that typically occurs. As Holland (2001) pointed out, the difference between trying to access these memories with and without the assistance of MDMA

> is that instead of feeling vulnerable and anxious during this experience, the patients remain relaxed, nearly fearless, and show a stronger sense of self and purpose. Feelings of depression and anxiety are replaced with a sense of ease and satiety. . . . An added and unexpected effect of MDMA is its potential pain killing property. Terminal patients who had been in chronic pain found themselves pain-free for the duration of the MDMA session. Adam earned the reputation of being "penicillin for the soul" and a "psychic pain-reliever": it offered healing to all who partook. (p. 2)

Anxiety is a major contributor to the experience of pain. Given that MDMA eliminates anxiety, this may be what is behind its analgesic properties.

General Effects

It takes about 30 to 45 minutes for MDMA to take effect. Some initial anxiety may be evoked by the experience of a slight feeling of drunkenness or shift in consciousness. This experience is accompanied by an intense feeling of euphoria and alertness. The client may explore objects and sounds, all of which bring pleasurable sensations and feelings of contentment. People are perceived as welcome contacts and as being immediately accepted, and the one feels emotional closeness with them. After this initial experience, the effects may decline slightly, but the client continues to accept their feelings and those of others. This self-acceptance of the totality of one's feelings can be deeply healing to people who are traumatized because it is the avoidance and negation of feelings that maintain PTSD. They are able to directly experience and communicate feelings related to traumatic events without camouflaging or minimizing them. During this plateau phase, which may last 2 to 3 hours, the client may feel other effects, such as a desire to move about, nystagmus, and jaw clenching (Holland, 2001). After about 3 hours, the effects begin to wane.

Some have reported that MDMA is a "love drug," and although MDMA may enhance the sense of touch, it can also make orgasms and erections more difficult to achieve, given the vasoconstrictive effects. For these reasons, it might be more appropriately called a "hug drug" (Holland, 2001) After about 6 hours following ingestion of MDMA, the effects are eliminated, but the experience of having confronted one's deep and formerly dreaded emotions and having accepted them continues. One may experience lingering feelings of headache, exhaustion, and possible mild insomnia. Over the next few days, the discussion with others about one's insights can further beneficially affect one's dealing with the traumatic experience. The literature (Mithoefer, Wagner, Mithoefer, Jerome, & Doblin, 2011) has reported little to no psychological regression or relapse from the beneficial psychological effects of MDMA.

An Individual Describes Their MDMA Experience

A regular user of MDMA and other mind-altering drugs reported the following experience to me. Although everyone's experience will be unique, this report is somewhat typical. The person described the MDMA experience in four stages.

During Stage 1, which lasts 20 to 60 minutes, one experiences an elevation of tension and perhaps anxiety. The energy level increases, accompanied by a desire to stretch, yawning, and jaw tightening. The sense of touch is altered such that a blanket or towel may produce an increased sense of pleasure and an overall pleasant sensation. The experience of "soft," for example, is enhanced and intensified. Colors and visual stimuli seem enhanced, as do auditory stimuli, especially music. One experiences a slight euphoria, a tingling, anxiety, and a clear elevation of the sense of heat and heart rate. The heart is "thumping." A sense of blissful euphoria then follows.

In Stage 2, which encompasses 1½ to 3 hours, one feels perfect contentment; a complete lack of insecurity; an absence of social anxiety; and a willingness to encounter, accept, and share their deepest feelings. A sense of "universal interconnectedness" follows and is accompanied by continuing euphoria. Auditory and tactile stimuli are "over the top pleasurable." The person encounters *nystagmus*, that is, involuntary eye movements or flicking, along with continued jaw tightening. Energy elevates, or, on the other extreme, one experiences a desire to "melt into the couch." Senses have elevated sensitivity, and music seems especially pleasurable.

Stage 3 lasts for a 1 hour to 2 hours and involves a slow and gradual waning of the effects from Stage 2. At high dosage levels, one may experience visual distortions and other visual effects, such as seeing an object and then, when looking again, noticing it is not there. Based on my observations from interviews, such experiences are transient and soon forgotten given the overall pleasant feelings while taking MDMA.

Stage 4 includes an "afterglow" effect: The person is in a good mood and feels positive for the next few days. However, if one has taken too much MDMA, one instead might feel a negative or depressive mood that can last for days or even weeks. Unless one "respects the drug" and takes it wisely, they will be punished by the crash experience. If a person takes the correct amount, about 80 to 130 micrograms, they will find that they are able to forgive themselves for whatever has taken place during the drug experience.

MDMA and Other Psychoactive Drugs

The MDMA experience differs for individuals as a function of their intentions, preparation, and environment in which the drugs are taken. Those who take the drug for party purposes will describe a different experience versus those who take it for psychotherapeutic or spiritual exploration purposes. MDMA is unique among the psychoactive drugs in that it is called an *entactogen*, which means "to touch within" (Nichols, 1986), or an *empathogen*, emphasizing an enhanced ability to empathize with oneself or others. Under the influence of MDMA, one wants to experience their feelings and share feelings with others. This desire to experience rather than avoid feelings can serve a therapeutic purpose, especially with regard to the treatment of PTSD in which the sufferer most often desires to avoid painful feelings.

Drugs like LSD are considered hallucinogens because they produce a variety of hallucinatory experiences. Narcotics like heroin produce tranquility and stupor, and amphetamine-like substances produce energy and mood elevation. Empathogens produce a feeling of tranquility, peace, and gentleness, as well as feelings of closeness, empathy, and a new awareness of the significance of music. Based on my interviews, users of empathogens have reported feelings of joy and an awareness of the importance of interpersonal relationships and relations with the self, and loss of self-consciousness along with of a sense of lack of the importance of time. Some encounter a spiritual awakening along with a universal insight and appreciation and love of all things.

Side Effects

A clear difference emerges between the effects of MDMA when used for psychotherapeutic or spiritual purposes versus when overused for party purposes; use of MDMA is far less problematic than overuse at a party or rave. Problems involving side effects are seldom reported when MDMA is used therapeutically. When taken at high levels and repeatedly in the rave and club scenes, one faces the danger of significant elevation of body temperature (hyperthermia) and dehydration, which leads some people to drink large amounts of liquids and experience a resulting electrolyte imbalance and possible brain swelling. These dehydration and overheating effects are enhanced by the activity level and close body contact in rave venues. Normally, when body temperature elevates, the response is to reduce activity. But the stimulant properties of MDMA, when taken in a party atmosphere, can result in increased physical activity. Body temperatures as high as 109 °F can cause organ failure, such as brain swelling or liver and kidney failure, which can be fatal (Henry & Rella, 2001; Holland, 2001). However, the number of reported deaths from MDMA is far fewer than that seen from smoking, alcohol abuse, or even over-the-counter medications (Lachenmeier & Rehm, 2015).

MDMA significantly elevates heart rate and can reduce the pumping efficiency of the heart in people who use it regularly. Regular usage can also reduce the desirable effects of MDMA, which leads to increasing the dosage level. People often report restless legs, illogical or disorganized thoughts, nausea, hot flashes or chills, headache, sweating, and muscle or joint stiffness. Increased and impulsive sexual activity stemming from the desire to make contact with others increases the chances of acquiring socially transmitted diseases. The week following overuse of MDMA can eventuate in depression, impaired attention and memory, anxiety, aggression, and irritability (Lachenmeier & Rehm, 2015).

Although somewhat rare, MDMA can produce *serotonin syndrome*, which results from excess release of this neurochemical. The syndrome is characterized by increased sweating, confusion, trouble walking, diarrhea, jerking muscles, erratic control of blood pressure and heart rate, muscle rigidity and increased muscle tone; this syndrome can lead to hyperthermia and result in death (Ames & Wirshing, 1993; Holland, 2001). The multitude of negative reports resulting from abuse of MDMA is what resulted in the federal banning of the drug. However, the positive reports of its psychotherapeutic utility in dealing with the characteristically treatment-resistant condition of PTSD served as a stimulus for its reconsideration as a therapeutic agent.

Clinical Trials of MDMA

MDMA is currently undergoing FDA clinical trials to determine its utility and safety in treating PTSD and related trauma disorders, and is in Phase III of these trials (Multidisciplinary Association for Psychedelic Studies [MAPS], n.d.). In Phase I, a small group of healthy volunteers take MDMA to determine its safety profile and how it might be used in the body. In Phase II, a large group of volunteers who have PTSD takes carefully measured doses. An objective assessment is made of how well the potential medicine treats or prevents the PTSD and provides a more extensive safety evaluation. In Phase III, hundreds and, in some cases, thousands of individuals are evaluated. This group includes a diverse mix of age, sex, race, and other demographics, all of whom are diagnosed with PTSD. One goal of Phase III trials is to identify side effects that might be seen in any of the samples or subsamples of participants. A second goal is to compare the new medicine with existing treatments and further evaluate its safety and efficacy profile in treating whatever it is intended to treat. Some expect MDMA to be approved for trauma treatment in the early 2020s (MAPS, n.d.).

Description of Mechanism of Action

The neurobiological effects of MDMA are fairly complex, involving various brain structures, neurochemicals, and modes of action. In this section, I present an overview for the benefit of clinicians.

   The experiential impact of MDMA results, in part, from its effects on two brain neurotransmitters: serotonin and dopamine. MDMA stimulates the release of serotonin and also inhibits the reuptake of this neurotransmitter; the overall result is an excess of serotonin in the nervous system. MDMA also causes a dopamine release comparatively less than that of serotonin (Holland, 2001). In addition, it suppresses monoamine oxidase, which can break down neurochemicals. These combined actions lead to an elevation of neurochemicals involved in nerve cell transmission.

   MDMA also elevates the hormones oxytocin and prolactin. Oxytocin is associated with increases in the desire for affiliation. Prolactin produces feelings of relaxation and a sense of satisfaction. MDMA has been associated with a quieting of the amygdala, that subcortical brain structure that mediates anxiety and the fight–flight–freeze response. MDMA can mimic the effects of Prozac (fluoxetine), the selective serotonin reuptake inhibitor, while also stimulating the release of serotonin and dopamine. It is interesting that those who take Prozac or other selective serotonin reuptake inhibitors like Paxil (paroxetine) or Zoloft (sertraline) for depression may experience a diminished effect of MDMA in that MDMA and these antidepressants use similar sites and mechanisms of action, and one tends to blunt or supplant the other (Holland, 2001). Similarly, when taken in combination with LSD, MDMA can have a mellowing effect on LSD, again because of a reputed competition for neurochemical releasing and reuptake sites. The process of combining MDMA and

LSD is referred to as "candy flipping" and is said to result in hallucinogenic experiences that are both toned down and accompanied by feelings of empathy and euphoria. These drug combinations have not been scientifically vetted in terms of any possible psychotherapeutic effect on such problems as PTSD. The FDA Phase III trials (MAPS, n.d.) mentioned earlier are meant to investigate the therapeutic effects of MDMA itself and not in combination with other drugs. Nevertheless, it is worth noting that MAPS (2014b) is in the process of evaluating the efficacy of marijuana in treating PTSD and has been awarded a grant of over $2 million by the State of Colorado to do so. MDMA studies are much further along in terms of investigating its effectiveness in treating PTSD.

Typical MDMA Therapy Session for Treating PTSD

It is difficult to overstate the value found in MDMA for those with treatment-resistant PTSD. In many of the empirical studies I present later, individuals may have been suffering from PTSD for decades and tried every known therapy, but they have been unable to overcome the disorder. The well-regarded MAPS, along with other like-minded organizations, has supported the research studies for MDMA and other psychedelic drugs, as have private donors.

The typical MDMA session is not the usual 45-minutes-to-1-hour psychotherapy office visit but usually lasts 8 or more hours during drug-supported treatment and may occur over 3 days spaced 2 to 6 weeks apart. The therapy involves an experienced pair of therapists: one male and one female. It is important to have therapists of different genders participating for empathic purposes. For instance, if the client's PTSD was a result of sexual assault by a male, it would be beneficial to have a female present, and if combat was the source of PTSD, a male presence could help. Eight to 16 weeks of additional non-MDMA sessions follow, each session often lasting 90 minutes. Before beginning the MDMA treatment, the therapists fully explain expected effects to lower the client's anxiety level. This explanatory or preparatory stage often encompasses two sessions and is always important in psychotherapy, but is especially so in cases in which one is dealing with traumatic experiences and the attendant anxiety that confronting these experiences characteristically evokes.

Once the therapists have addressed the client's questions and concerns are addressed, they give the trauma victim a dose of MDMA of 100 mg to 125 mg with the expectation that approximately 90 minutes later, the client will receive another dose of about half that amount to enhance the experience. In experimental studies, a control group with an active placebo can be used. An active placebo is needed because there would be no way for a true placebo control group to be unaware of their active–inactive status, given that the impact of MDMA is so obvious. The active placebo is usually a dose of approximately 40 mg of MDMA.

The male–female therapist team provides support, answers questions, and typically pursues a nondirective, reflective approach during the session. This is similar to the procedure that takes place in an eye-movement desensitization and reprocessing (EMDA) session in which the therapist tries not to guide the trauma victim but simply asks nondirective questions, such as "What came up next?" or "What did you then experience?" The nondirective approach is used because every client has their own narrative and way of viewing and understanding what their experiences are. It is desirable to have therapists who are familiar with treating trauma and have training in such areas as cognitive behavior therapy (CBT), exposure, desensitization, transference, and countertransference. There is no "correct" way of seeing one's trauma experiences. Often three such sessions occur with therapists filling the role of mutual collaborators or participants who go through the trauma experiences and associated emotions with the client. The two therapists and the trauma victim embark on a mutual experience of encountering what took place during the trauma and all associated feelings attached to it. Three 8-hour sessions are not a practical means of treatment for most clinicians. As a result, many would consider such an approach a last resort for those whose PTSD or trauma experiences have been treatment resistant for many years.

In an attempt to dissociate or disconnect from trauma experiences, trauma sufferers also disconnect from themselves. It is impossible to disconnect from part of one's own experience without disconnecting from what makes up one's identity. What transpires within the MDMA session is a complete acceptance of, rather than a disconnection from, the trauma and all associated emotions, and in that way, a person comes to a full acceptance of themselves. Trauma ceases to be the sole focus of the session, but, rather, the whole person with all associated feelings, thoughts, behaviors, intentions and expectations are accepted nonjudgmentally. Trauma is no longer cut off; instead, it is integrated into the selfhood of the person. All descriptions of the trauma become part of the emotional makeup of the individual, and all emotions are welcome and dealt with in an environment of a complete absence of anxiety and fear. A new awareness and acceptance of the self—all aspects of the self—begin to develop.

As in EMDR, the healing process continues over time. Twelve-month follow-up studies (e.g., Mithoefer et al., 2013) show continuing reductions of scores on standardized trauma measures. It appears as if the body and mind (or "bodymind," to use Candace Pert's, 1999, term) wants to move in the direction of healing. Just as superficial wounds heal over time and don't normally "un-heal," the emotional repair brought about by the use of MDMA continues over time, and little-to-no undoing that takes place. MDMA is not in itself a curative agent but appears to be more of a psychotherapeutic facilitator. It allows the trauma victim to welcome their unpleasant experiences without fear and avoidance, and once this welcoming and greeting of all aspects of one's life is experienced; the healing process is automatically set into motion.

Reports of those who have gone through MDMA sessions to treat trauma resemble epiphanies. In their prior lives, these clients had walled off painful experiences and were negatively impacted by these experiences. Anxiety, depression, and a gloomy perspective of the world and themselves were their way of going about daily life. After MDMA therapy, individuals have reported rediscovering themselves, accepting themselves totally, and finding a joy in living (Bravo, 2001). It is not an exaggeration to say that these newly treated individuals have had a spiritual awakening. Life becomes worth living. Trust, caring, and empathy replace fear and depression. The MDMA therapy experience is reported to be transformative and a kind of rebirth into a new, far more fulfilling way of being.

Specific Aspects of the Psychotherapy Used in MDMA Treatment for PTSD

The treatment approach used in an MDMA-assisted psychotherapy session is primarily nondirective and, as such, does not follow the traditionally used methods for treating PTSD, including the use of CBT and prolonged exposure. A treatment manual (MAPS, 2014a) is supplemented by training and evaluation of therapist skills (Mithoefer, 2017). A nondirective approach emphasizes invitation rather than direction. The approach respects and gives attention to one's unique modes of functioning, and this approach is commonly seen in methods like EMDR, acupuncture, and EFT. That mode of treatment emphasizes the body's and psyche's natural inclination to heal if provided with the correct circumstances. MDMA-assisted therapy seeks to provide those circumstances by encouraging exploration of experiences that arise from use of MDMA.

Providing a sense of safety and well-being is critical in MDMA-assisted therapy, given that the client will be directly dealing with experiences that have radically altered their lives in a negative way. Thus, the therapeutic alliance and trust are essential elements. The nondirective approach does not preclude guidance or redirection, which are used only to facilitate the participant's processing. The therapy should enhance processing rather than avoidance of aversive experiences, but should do so with respect for recognition that, at times, some level of avoidance may be necessary for the client to further manage and deal with their experiences. In those instances in which clients choose to avoid and resist processing, the therapists should facilitate and encourage curiosity on the client's part as to why they have moved to resistance and avoidance. "Therapists," stated Mithoefer (2017), "seek to maximize the benefits of inner experience catalyzed by MDMA, while at the same time ensuring that the participant is safe and is not re-traumatized by internal conflicts that may arise" (p. 8).

One male and one female therapist engage in empathic listening, which means that the therapists are nonjudgmental and offer the opportunity for clients to talk openly and honestly about their experience without concern over how the therapists might receive this experience. The goal is to allow clients freedom to express what they are experiencing and to have the comfort and confidence to know their therapists will accept and not evaluate what the client is reporting. The therapists' empathic presence involves delighting and rejoicing in the client's accomplishments and communicating that appreciation (Mithoefer, 2017). Empathic listeners are relaxed but engaged, asking questions and exploring without prying. The listener maintains appropriate eye contact and offers reassuring, appropriate touches if culturally acceptable and agreed to by participants. And, as Mithoefer (2017) pointed out, "Empathic listeners are not hesitant to admit they don't have answers" (p. 9).

The tempo of the session should unfold at a pace that is spontaneous for the client. Therapists must be tolerant and not attempt to move the client forward unless it becomes clear that some level of avoidance is taking place. Even then, it would be more desirable for the client to come to the realization that they are avoiding certain unpleasant experiences. Offering direction that is oriented toward facilitating the recognition of avoidance is permissible in those instances in which the client may be stuck and unable to see beyond their self-created roadblocks. In these situations, questions such as, "Why do you think this seems to be difficult for you?" are entirely appropriate in the nondirective approach because they are noninterpretive and not embedded in a particular psychotherapeutic orientation. Such questions are oriented toward fostering self-exploration and self-directed healing. This nondirective approach communicates a general sense of permission, receptivity, allowance, and acceptance of whatever comes from within the PTSD sufferer. On their part, therapists must be willing to surrender their adherence to didactic and directive modes of therapy in which they have been trained.

Therapists must trust that any trauma memories that continue to arise are occurring so the client can completely understand and process them, and begin to heal (Mithoefer, 2017). Therapists must have faith in a self-healing process of body and psyche, and their role is to present a safe, secure, emotionally facilitative environment in which this self-healing process can take place. It is important for therapists who engage in MDMA-assisted therapy to have training in treating trauma. Often this training is in areas such as CBT, EMDR, family systems therapy, psychodynamic psychotherapy, and trauma-focused CBT. It is sometimes a difficult transition to move from formal modes of training to one in which the therapy is guided not by theoretical orientation but by the client's inner experiences. Training may be needed though reading treatment manuals, watching videos, role-playing, and attendance at training sessions provided by organizations like MAPS. It may be that those trained in Eastern traditions may have an easier time with the nondirective approach than those trained in Western approaches having a directive focus. The goal is to present a supportive, accepting, and safe atmosphere in which inner-directed growth can take place.

Specific Aspects of the Therapy Setting

The therapeutic setting for MDMA, like the process of MDMA-assisted psychotherapy itself, requires an adjustment. The traditional therapist's office with a comfortable chair or couch is replaced by what might resemble a small den. In MDMA-assisted therapy, the room needs to be quiet and free from interruption. A futon or similar type of furniture should be available for the client to recline on or sit in, and pillows should be provided for support. Blankets are made available. One should allow room for two chairs so that the cotherapists can sit on either side of the futon. The room should be aesthetically pleasing with fresh flowers and tasteful artwork, and it needs to be a neat but comfortable environment that looks nothing like a hospital room. The space would benefit from an eating area and provision of easily digested food per the client's preferences. Client's should be informed that ready medical access is available in the unlikely event of any medical complications. This information is provided for both reasons of safety and to assure the client that they will be safe under all circumstances (Mithoefer, 2017).

The setting should include well-furnished sleeping arrangements so the client may spend the night after the session. If desired, accommodations can also be made for a spouse or partner to share the sleeping space. The therapists should discuss the client's preferences regarding snacks and liquids in advance, although those taking MDMA often have a reduced desire to eat. Electrolyte types of beverages should be provided because MDMA often produces body temperature elevation and a desire to drink. The therapists need to limit these liquids to about 3 liters per day to prevent hypernatremia, an overabundance of sodium in the blood. Snacks, such as crackers, should be available. Stereo equipment and music choices are made available because music is often used to encourage relaxation and self-reflection. The music frequently starts in a relaxing and calming fashion, and then engages in a succession of more active and emotionally arousing themes, followed by a quieter more meditative theme. Instrumental, as opposed to music with lyrics, is preferred. Therapists should prepare multi-hour playlists. Headphones are offered, and eyeshades are provided to assist in the process of inward searching.

Demands on Therapists

Conducting MDMA therapy can be demanding on therapists. Aside from receiving specialized training and developing competence in this type of therapy, therapists must provide time for sessions that prepare the client for the MDMA experience. They should decide what physical distance from each other during sessions is comfortable for them both, and they also need to be attuned to any changes in the client's comfort level with their physical proximity (Mithoefer, 2017). Therapists must discuss with the client that they may provide physical assistance and touch to help increase comfort level or even to serve as a form of resistance that the client may wish to push up against. No sexual contact of any kind is permitted. These discussions and agreements become necessary because those reencountering traumatic memories may be particularly vulnerable to feelings of being hurt or confined. The two therapists agree to remain with the client throughout the MDMA session, which can last for a full day. A therapist may leave the room, as needed, but at all times, at least one therapist available. Therapists and participants come to an agreement that after each MDMA-assisted session, they will have daily telephone contact for up to a week (Mithoefer, 2017). Therapists agree to be available 24 hours a day during this period. Therapists should be willing to accept that they may need to be available to clients for even longer periods if it is beneficial to and needed by the PTSD sufferer.

Clearly, the demands on therapists during MDMA-assisted therapy sessions and even before and after completion of sessions are considerable. This level of commitment is often willingly offered by those with a deep interest in trauma treatment and by those who know that they, too, will grow along with the client, because the client is overcoming traumas that have shackled them client for a lifetime. Nevertheless, therapists should have access to colleagues or other mental health professionals given that the demands on them are considerable and might lead to emotional exhaustion. Therapist burnout may be a possibility in those situations in which they have made a commitment to multiple MDMA sessions. Countering the possibility of burnout is that therapists who engage in this form of intervention are often inspired and fulfilled by the opportunity to watch, participate in, and share in the breakthroughs made by those who have suffered from the burdens of PTSD, frequently for decades.

Scientific Studies of MDMA

The first randomized controlled study comparing MDMA-assisted psychotherapy for 20 clients with treatment-resistant PTSD against a placebo (Mithoefer et al., 2011) provided hard data on the efficacy of MDMA therapy. These clients had received both psychotherapy and psychopharmacology over the years for their PTSD but had shown no improvement. Compared with 25% of the placebo group, 83% of those in the MDMA psychotherapy group no longer met the criteria for PTSD after 16 psychotherapy sessions in which MDMA was administered three times. Both groups received an equal number and duration of sessions but the placebo group did not receive MDMA. A follow-up (Mithoefer et al., 2013) to this study was conducted 4 years later, and more than 80% of the MDMA group continued to no longer meet PTSD criteria. In other words, little relapse was shown.

That follow-up study (Mithoefer et al., 2013), which had 19 participants, used standardized measures such as the Clinician-Administered PTSD Scale (Blake et al., 1990), the Impact of Event Scale (Horowitz, Wilner, & Alvarez, 1979), and others, that are psychometrically valid and reliable. In addition, the authors included several physiological measures, such as heart rate, blood pressure, and body temperature, along with a number of body chemistry assessments. Every effort was made to treat the MDMA and placebo group similarly. Two, 90-minute introductory sessions were conducted within 6 weeks of the start of therapy. Then the formal treatment sessions took place and lasted for 8 to 10 hours, plus study participants spent the night at the treatment clinic. A male and female therapist who were nondirective in their approach attended the treatment sessions and encouraged participants to allow themselves to experience whatever thoughts, feelings, and perceptions arose in response to treatment. After the extended treatment sessions, the authors conducted pre- and postassessments with psychological and physiological measures. The next day, they conducted another 90-minute session and then provided daily phone calls for a week.

In the MDMA group, participants were given 125 mg of the drug, and between 2 and 2½ hours later, a half dose of 62.5 mg was provided (Mithoefer et al., 2013). Onset of effects of MDMA occurred 45 to 75 minutes after the initial dose and lasted 4 to 5 hours. Several physical symptoms were noted primarily in the MDMA group, including elevation in pulse rate, blood pressure, and body temperature. Also noted in the MDMA group were jaw tightness, nausea, a feeling of being cold, dizziness, loss of appetite, and impaired balance. Overall, the MDMA group showed highly significant and positive changes on measures associated with improvements in PTSD symptoms in comparison with the placebo group. Placebo participants were later offered MDMA treatment because they, like the MDMA group, had significant PTSD problems at the start of the study. Those control participants who then took MDMA showed similar improvements as the MDMA treatment group. The authors viewed their results as promising but cited study limitations, including small sample size and that those in the placebo group probably were aware of their assignment because of the pronounced effects seen in the MDMA group and the lack of those effects for placebo participants.

Placebo Effects Issues

Placebo effects can be both beneficial and problematic. They are helpful in that the mere expectancy of improvement can have beneficial effects in producing both imagined and real improvements. When medications are compared with placebos, such as sugar pills, the magnitude of the difference between the medication and the sugar pill represents the actual impact of the medication independent of the expectancy for improvement. In such studies comparing active medications with placebos (e.g., Mithoefer et al., 2011), it is often surprising to find that the medically inert placebo actually results in improvements. Some have speculated that the expectancy for change enhances the immune system and thus results in positive changes. Recall that certain arthroscopic knee surgery procedures and sham arthroscopic procedures frequently show no difference in effectiveness (see Chapter 7 in this volume). Both show improvement. This finding can be interpreted as either that placebos produce an effect equivalent to actual surgery or that neither approach was effective, and that the natural healing process, along with exercise, is what accounted for improvement in both the real and sham surgery. Regardless of which interpretation is valid, it is clear that although placebo effects can be beneficial, they complicate the interpretation of findings. Such was the case in the Mithoefer et al. (2011) study.

"Active" Placebo

In the Mithoefer et al. (2011) study, it was not possible to compare the MDMA intervention with a placebo because it appeared to be a real possibility that those in the placebo group knew their group assignment. Those in the placebo condition did not experience the distinct physiological and psychological effects expected by those taking MDMA. To combat this problem, what is needed is a study using an "active" placebo that mimics the physical and psychological effects of MDMA.

Such a study was conducted by Oehen, Traber, Widmer, and Schnyder (2013). Like the Mithoefer et al. (2011) study, this one also used a dosage of 125 mg followed by a second half dosage 2.5 hours later of 62.5 mg. This stage of the study, Stage 1, unlike the Mithoefer et al. (2011) study, included an active placebo of 37.5 mg given to a second group of traumatized participants. This dose was chosen because it was expected it would not result in a significant increase in anxiety or produce unwanted upsetting memories of trauma, although the dose was expected to yield slight alterations of perception and increase in relaxation. By using the 37.5 mg of MDMA, the placebo control participants would be less able to determine whether they were in the experimental or control group because they, too, were experiencing sensations and perceptions that would normally be expected of MDMA.

In Stage 2 of the study, after sufficient data were collected using psychometrically valid and reliable measures, those in the active placebo condition were offered engagement in the full MDMA experimental condition. In Stage 3 of the study, those who did not show a sufficient response to the full MDMA dose were given a dose of 150 mg and a supplemental dose of 75 mg. Three sessions of MDMA administration, including full and half dosages, were conducted over a period of weeks. In addition, participants were provided with 12 non-drug therapy sessions that were interspersed between MDMA sessions.

Overall findings of the study (Oehen et al., 2013) were that the full MDMA group experienced significant reductions in self-reported PTSD symptoms in comparison with the control group but not on one of the standardized measures of PTSD (i.e., Clinician-Administered PTSD Scale; Blake et al., 1990). What this means is that even at the lower dosage level given to the active placebo group, positive effects of MDMA plus psychotherapy occurred. In addition, the authors found that three MDMA sessions were more effective than two. A follow-up study conducted a year later (Mithoefer et al., 2013) showed that the reductions in PTSD symptoms were maintained, and the study authors found even further reductions on the Clinician-Administered PTSD Scale. Other studies have shown maintenance of improvements over a period of several years. This study (Mithoefer et al., 2013), together with the Mithoefer et al. (2011) study, shows that MDMA-assisted therapy can significantly reduce PTSD symptoms in a treatment-resistant group, including those who have tried a wide spectrum of therapies over a period of decades. There were no noticeable negative side effects that followed from the MDMA intervention.

Cautionary Statements

Despite the positive findings regarding MDMA treatment for PTSD, it is important to consider that these improvements cannot be attributed to the use of MDMA alone. If this were the case, all that would be required to heal the millions of PTSD sufferers throughout the world would be to encourage them to take MDMA or even Ecstasy, and their problems would disappear. The studies that have been done or are in the process of being conducted involve the administration of pure MDMA, rather than the often adulterated Ecstasy found in the party and street scene, and the drug administration is accompanied by intensive psychotherapy. The MDMA used in research studies is given under carefully supervised and controlled conditions with available medical access, and is accompanied by, most importantly, psychotherapy. None of the research presented in the literature involves MDMA administration without psychotherapy. The psychotherapy used in these studies is oriented toward providing a supportive, security-enhancing environment along with gentle guidance focused on helping the client confront and deal with experiences that once produced extremes of fear and avoidance.

In addition, the psychotherapy provided in MDMA studies involves male–female therapy teams, which can certainly add to the cost of treatment. However, if one compares the cost of decades of psychotherapy for treatment-resistant cases of PTSD, the male–female therapy team approach, even with multiple sessions, might still be the more cost-effective way to go. Additional research involving MDMA treatment for PTSD might be able to streamline treatment procedures and reduce costs. The traditionally used medications for PTSD, Zoloft (sertraline) and Paxil (paroxetine) appear to not only be less effective than MDMA but also require ongoing medication management and daily dosing. Thousands of accidental and intentional overdoses of these selective serotonin reuptake inhibitors and the dangers of other commonly used prescription drugs, such as benzodiazepines, other hypnotics, mood stabilizers, and antipsychotics, cannot be overestimated. In contrast, MDMA is administered in a clinical setting with no take-home doses (Feduccia, Holland, & Mithoefer, 2018) and, as such, presents few dangers of side effects, abuse, or self-harm.

Status of Empirical Support

The empirical support for the effectiveness of MDMA in treating highly treatment-resistant cases of PTSD is impressive. It is for this reason that the FDA has granted this drug "breakthrough" status and is fully in support of further investigations of its efficacy. The therapeutic procedure of treating PTSD with MDMA is both labor and time intensive. However, when one considers that many cases of treatment for PTSD can last for decades and not be all that effective, MDMA-assisted psychotherapy may offer an overall savings in time, resources, and the lessening of suffering. It is clearly an alternative therapy for PTSD that appears to be both novel and highly effective.

SUMMARY

As of this writing, the FDA is overseeing Phase III trials in which relatively large numbers of traumatized individuals are participating in randomized double blind, placebo-controlled studies. Emerging results of these studies appear promising. Problematically, MDMA continues to be considered a Schedule I substance, and as a result, its possession and distribution are illegal, which can deter active investigations of the drug. Despite its sanctioned status, it is a drug that can have real benefit to large numbers of people. The major value of MDMA-assisted therapy may be that it creates a psychological and biomedical environment in which trauma sufferers are able to confront their trauma memories and experiences again without the extreme anxiety and reflexive avoidance that occurs without this drug. It is well known in the world of trauma therapy that one overcomes their traumatic experiences by processing them through higher brain centers. The extreme levels of anxiety that this potential processing entails forecloses this avenue of treatment to many PTSD sufferers. MDMA effectively removes that roadblock and, as such, has an impressive capability of bringing about cures.

It is likely that once further studies of MDMA-assisted therapy are conducted, the complexity of treatment can be streamlined, which will allow such treatments to be more accessible to increasing numbers of trauma sufferers. But even if such streamlining does not occur, this form of therapy is still a major advance in treatment. Another possibility is that with further research, it may be determined that MDMA-assisted therapy will prove beneficial in the treatment of other common psychological disorders in addition to trauma and PTSD. MDMA, despite its unfortunate and problematic association with the rave and club scene, appears to be on the verge, as of this writing, of earning an important place among those valuable alternative therapies for PTSD.

10

Key Takeaways and Other Alternative Therapies

The development of posttraumatic stress disorder (PTSD) can be and often is a life-changing event. It creates a self significantly altered from the pretrauma self who is, in some ways, unrecognizable. A few years ago, I was told of a young man who killed his psychiatrist. The psychiatric sessions frequently turned into occasions for sexual abuse of the young client. When questioned, the young man is said to have stated that he got to the point at which he didn't know who the hell he was anymore and just wanted to stop what was going on. The abuse was deeply traumatizing and appeared to change this youth from a feeling and hurt being into an animal under attack that feared for the loss of its world and which then attacked in response because of a need to survive. PTSD victims frequently report feeling dehumanized and animalized. Rape victims often feel "thing-a-fied," meaning they are altered from a human being with a full spectrum of emotions into a frightened thing on whom sexual and aggressive behaviors have been meted out. They wind up feeling less human and more objectlike. This self-change is deep and confusing to the PTSD victim.

My own experience was a transformation from a thoughtful, conscientious young man into a wary animal. This animal trusted no one and deeply felt that the community and environment were dangerous, and this feeling created a need to be constantly on guard. Survival was all that mattered. Now, these descriptions of PTSD are certainly problematic, but what makes them

http://dx.doi.org/10.1037/0000186-011
Alternative Therapies for PTSD: The Science of Mind–Body Treatments, by R. W. Motta

even more disturbing is that the negative changes to self can persist for many years, and sometimes a lifetime.

ENDURANCE OF PTSD

Why are the changes so deep and long lasting? Even the death of a loved one eventually results in acceptance and moving on, although doing so can sometime take years. Most other troubling events, such as relationship breakups, fender-bender car accidents, interpersonal conflicts, and work stresses, can be seriously troubling and upsetting but don't cause self-changes that persist for years. The reason why PTSD is so altering is that one encounters experiences so extreme and so disruptive that they cause a reframing or reconceptualization of one's world. Whereas previously one may have had core beliefs like "good deeds pay off," "honesty is the best policy," or "integrity matters," they now question all of those core views because they see that the world is not fair or just, that it is a jungle that values wariness, being on guard, and being prepared for attack to survive.

To overcome PTSD, two things must take place. First, the sufferer has to revisit those experiences that produced the trauma and try to understand them objectively and with intelligence and perspective. This is a remarkably difficult task, and the more typical response is to not revisit but rather to avoid. Second, they then have to take a leap of faith involving letting their guard down incrementally and starting to trust again. Both of these tasks are extremely difficult, to say the least. How does one again confront those experiences that caused such extreme levels of fear and life threat? Attempts to do so, to wade back into the waters that produced such extreme fear, are virtually impossible for perhaps the majority of those with PTSD. Why? Because these efforts produce extreme fear even to the level of the fear of annihilation. Once this confronting takes place and the fear begins to subside, then one begins to let down their guard, reintegrate themselves into society, and begin to trust their world. Letting down the very defenses that one believes kept them alive— kept them surviving—is not an easy thing to do.

It is for these reasons that treating PTSD is so difficult. As soon as the therapist begins to get close to the traumatic experiences, the client is often so flooded with fear that they leave the therapy session, never to return. All trauma therapists have experienced this disturbing outcome. The standard tools, the "gold standard" cognitive behavior therapy (CBT)-type therapies, are helpful only for those who stay in therapy. Unfortunately, a minority of clients stays with trauma therapy. It is simply too upsetting and too difficult to tolerate. Therapists need alternative approaches that don't create such a reflexive fear response. Many of the alternative treatment approaches presented in this book are designed to help clinicians bring their clients along from fearful isolated existences into a world they once knew and have long since fled from.

STRENGTHS AND WEAKNESSES IN THE APPLICATION OF ALTERNATIVE THERAPIES FOR PTSD

Each of the alternative approaches I have covered gives therapists an additional tool for managing and treating PTSD. Each approach is valuable but not without limitations. These limitations are typically not weaknesses of the procedures per se but in the professional resistance to their use and acceptance.

Eye-Movement Desensitization and Reprocessing

Strengths

One strength of eye-movement desensitization and reprocessing (EMDR) is that it does not demand that one directly confront their trauma but rather the images that may be associated with that trauma. It also does not call on the therapist to push the client to confront again their trauma experiences but instead to query them about what associations come up after each series of alternating eye (or other) movements. It is a client-directed approach. Another strength is that progress appears to be resistant to relapse, and relapse is a common problem with traditional approaches to PTSD treatment. In addition, it has been scientifically vetted and accepted as an empirically supported treatment by many major professional organizations, such as the American Psychological Association, World Health Organization, and International Society for Traumatic Stress Studies.

Weaknesses

A possible weakness of EMDR is that despite its acceptance by professional organizations and the abundance of studies supporting its effectiveness in treating trauma, many continue consider it akin to voodoo and as pseudoscience. This view is unfortunate, and it clearly reveals the entrenchment of traditional ideas and resistance to new ones. CBT is primarily based on widely accepted principles of learning. In contrast, the theoretical basis of EMDR's utility remains unclear. Some claim that it involves information-processing alterations; others claim that it results in functional neurological changes. Its difficulty fitting into traditional explanations for its mechanisms of action cause many to unjustly reject it as little more than exposure or simply the result of placebo effects. Perhaps a further weakness is that EMDR is a fairly complex process involving multiple phases and methods of assessment. It requires some degree of training and should not be attempted by anyone who is not also trained as a clinician.

Yoga

Strengths

One of the primary strengths of yoga is its ability to integrate body and mind though a series of stretches and postures. This is no small attainment for those suffering from PTSD because these individuals have separated out painful aspects of their experiences to avoid suffering. They frequently are out of touch with what their body is doing. This separation or "dis"-integration stands in the way of healing. Yoga practices produce a tying together or reintegration of one's emotional or cognitive self with one's physical self. Many well-designed empirical studies show that yoga practice significantly reduces PTSD symptoms. Another strength is that it is easily learned and does not require professional clinical training to administer or self-administer.

Weaknesses

A perceived weakness of yoga is that it is not seen as "real" therapy but rather as an Eastern medicine type of body practice that is good for physical flexibility and little else. My personal internist recently told me that he does yoga weekly "to stretch my muscles—not for any of those mystical reasons." That well-controlled studies support yoga as an intervention for PTSD is simply lost on many health care providers. An additional weakness of yoga may be that many people consider it to be a lifelong practice and not an intervention one does for a limited number of sessions, such as might occur in traditional psychotherapy. Yoga requires a long-term commitment that many may be unwilling to make.

Mindfulness Meditation

Strengths

The strength of mindfulness, like yoga, is that it is not a complex skill to learn but is one requiring dedication and practice. The dedicated practice of mindfulness can lead to a deep nonjudgmental acceptance of self and others. This self-acceptance and other acceptance are major problem areas for PTSD sufferers. The peace and tranquility brought about through continued meditation practice are completely novel and unexpected, especially for those suffering from PTSD. The norm for those with PTSD is to be on guard, on edge, and distrusting of others and of the environment. Mindfulness and yoga are practiced in the Veterans Health Administration, and combatants find it a valuable alternative to CBT and prolonged exposure (PE) approaches. Veterans seek out this mode of intervention, a testament to its utility and also a clear statement of the desire to avoid more traditional modes of intervention.

Weaknesses

Like other alternative therapies for PTSD, many health care providers do not see mindfulness as a "true" treatment of PTSD despite its wide acceptance. Another possible weakness of mindfulness may be that for it to have a major and long-lasting impact on the lives of PTSD sufferers, it must be practiced with a great deal of dedication or what I heard Kabat-Zinn call "sincerity of purpose" (at a conference). Practicing for 20 or so minutes daily for years is simply not something that most people are willing to do. Despite its benefits, many would prefer to take a tranquilizing pill to reduce their stress. They seldom consider that the tranquilizing pill produces a temporary and ephemeral respite and, in many instances, is contraindicated in trauma treatment. Many often choose immediate pain relief over the sustained relief that a dedicated meditation practice produces.

Exercise

Strengths

Many strengths are associated with exercise. It is not too far from the mark to say that exercise is something of an elixir for treating psychological and physical distress. Its elixir status is earned because of its ability to reduce PTSD, reduce anxiety and depression, reduce obsessive-compulsive disorder, reduce tics seen in Tourette's disorder, enhance self-esteem, improve concentration, improve cognitive skills and cognitive clarity, enhance perceptions of self-worth and self-efficacy, and improve one's sense of well-being and equanimity. And this is just a partial listing of its psychological benefits. Exercise also offers a myriad of physical benefits not within the scope of this discussion. Compared with traditional psychotherapy, it is low to no cost and does not require professionals to guide its use. It does not carry the stigma of being a "psychotherapy" and therefore is acceptable to many who might be otherwise averse to treatment.

Weaknesses

A drawback of exercise as an intervention for PTSD is that it is not seen as an "official" therapy, even though few official interventions have such a wide-ranging positive impact across so many domains. Another possible "weakness" of exercise is that it requires a good deal of discipline to do on a regular basis, and some people consider it unpleasant. Most people in the United States do little to no exercise despite knowing its benefits. In addition, many studies show that exercise in and of itself is at least comparable in effectiveness with medication and psychotherapy for many disorders, including those related to trauma. So, it not being considered an "official" therapy is both a strength to some and a weakness to others.

Nature- and Animal-Assisted Therapy

Strengths

The major strength of nature-assisted therapy (NAT) and animal-assisted therapy (AAT) is that they are both readily accessible to most PTSD sufferers and they almost completely negate any of the anxieties evoked from the confrontation of one's trauma experiences as seen in traditional therapy. Large numbers of combat veterans and troubled youths have benefited from being engaged with nature and involved with animals. Nature seems to enhance feelings of tranquility, and animals have the unique ability to allow individuals to get back in touch with feelings they have long abandoned or suppressed. Pets are viewed as unconditionally accepting and wanting to give and receive attention and affection. For the PTSD sufferer, pets are trusted, but humans are often a question mark.

Weaknesses

The perceived weakness of NAT and AAT is primarily that few see them as valid forms of intervention for alleviating symptoms of trauma. Even though they work toward humanizing those who have been dehumanized does not seem to enhance their being seen as valued treatment approaches to ameliorating the suffering of people with PTSD. The existence of empirically valid studies supporting the value of NAT and AAT in managing PTSD, as well as their popularity among many traumatized groups, seems to have had little impact on their credibility.

Acupuncture

Strengths

The strength of acupuncture is simply that is accepted worldwide for the treatment of various disorders and especially for those involving pain. Randomized, controlled, and blinded studies have found acupuncture to be an effective intervention for PTSD. It does not require confronting of traumatic experiences and is therefore far less likely to be rejected than are traditional psychotherapies for PTSD. It is a valuable tool for those looking for treatment alternatives for PTSD. Its value in treating a variety of disorders, both physical and psychological, is supported by the World Health Organization, and millions of people all over the world have satisfactorily used acupuncture.

Weaknesses

The weaknesses of acupuncture for PTSD are threefold. First, it requires a high degree of specialized training to develop expertise in the technique. Second, it requires multiple sessions within a specified period, so it may be costly and inconvenient for the PTSD sufferer. And third, its effectiveness, which is hard to question, appears to be based on nothing that can be substantiated by Western views. The effect of acupuncture is said to result from the unblocking of meridians through which an energy of qi flows. Western medicine cannot validate the existence of these meridians, their placement, or qi. Thus, many negate acupuncture as a "real" treatment of any disorder, whether physical or emotional, and view it as a dubious procedure despite its effectiveness.

Emotional Freedom Techniques

Strengths

The strength of emotional freedom techniques (EFT) is that they are easily taught and are self-help techniques that can be of value in treating a variety of emotional issues, including PTSD. A further strength is that EFT is based on the same principles as acupuncture and should be effective for the same reasons that acupuncture is, namely, blocking the flow of energy through the meridians.

Another strength is that it has received validation from well-controlled empirical studies.

Weaknesses

The inability of Western medicine to explain the effects of EFT results in doubts about its efficacy. However, EFT is based on the same line of reasoning for its effectiveness as is acupuncture, which, with the passage of time, has become more widely accepted than EFT. Little evidence in the West has been found for either meridians or of the energy that flows through these meridians. A further weakness of EFT is that it is "the new kid on the block." Any new procedure is likely to be met with resistance and skepticism. Acupuncture, reportedly used for centuries, has only recently received a degree of acceptance in the United States. EFT has a long road to travel before it reaches a similar level of acceptability, and even that level leaves a good deal to be desired. Its advocates claim that it has met the standards required to be an empirically validated treatment. Nevertheless, many probably consider it a "fringe" technique despite the scientific studies that support its use and efficacy.

MDMA ("Ecstasy")

Strengths

The major strength of MDMA (3,4-methylenedioxymethamphetamine) in treating PTSD is that it has been fast tracked by the U.S. Food and Drug Administration and awarded "breakthrough" status. It has shown itself to be highly effective in reducing the anxiety and avoidance that accompanies traumatic experiences. This reduction in fear allows the PTSD victim to confront and explore the issues surrounding their PTSD with a sense of curiosity and interest rather than of fear and avoidance. It is this ability to directly confront, process, and deal with the trauma that leads to dramatic improvements. The drug is referred to as an "empathogen" because of its ability to generate empathy for oneself and others. It is likely that MDMA will become a recognized and Food and Drug Administration–sanctioned drug for PTSD simply because numerous well-controlled studies have provided impressive evidence for its effectiveness, and these studies are fairly consistent in their findings. Many of the participants in these studies have been suffering from treatment-resistant PTSD for decades and have tried multiple forms of medical and psychological treatment to no avail. When enrolled in an MDMA trial, they often show remarkable improvements, and these positive changes don't seem to show much of, if any, relapse.

Weaknesses

The first obvious weakness of MDMA as a treatment for PTSD is that the drug is a Schedule I substance and thus is illegal for use or sale. It is an experimental drug and is unavailable except in clinical trials and in the rave and party scenes, where it is often adulterated and of unknown purity. A further weakness is that the therapeutic process involving MDMA treatment is cumbersome and requires two trained therapists, multiple all-day sessions, the availability of emergency medical support, and around-the-clock availability of psychological support throughout an extended treatment period involving nondrug sessions. All of this is costly. This weakness must, however, be put into perspective. If known traditional treatments for PTSD are used for many years, they can be hugely expensive and ultimately futile. MDMA, despite its cumbersome application process, may be comparatively cost-effective by comparison.

WHAT ABOUT OTHER ALTERNATIVE THERAPIES?

The alternative approaches to treating PTSD that I have presented up to this point are those that have garnered substantial empirical support and yet do not generate the high levels of anxiety that results from confronting trauma-related memories. I have not included full descriptions and analyses of the following alternative therapies for treating PTSD because they either (a) are very difficult to tolerate because of a tendency to evoke extreme anxiety and avoidance responses or (b) are comparatively lacking in compelling empirical support.

Virtual Reality Exposure Therapy

Virtual reality exposure therapy (VRET) is an alternative not covered because it is a variant of exposure therapy and, as such, is likely to produce strong avoidance responses in people with severe cases of PTSD. VRET typically involves a motion-tracked, head-mounted display that can be augmented with vibration, odors, sounds, medications, and physical props (e.g., rifles). It has been used extensively to treat PTSD related to wars in Vietnam, Afghanistan, and Iraq. Dropout rates are seldom reported in studies on this type of therapy. Also, little to no research shows that VRET is any more effective than traditional PE. The major difficulty with VRET is that it, like PE, evokes strong avoidance and extreme levels of anxiety in many who are the most traumatized. I have tried VRET and was able to tolerate it for fewer than 5 seconds. General agreement is that PE and perhaps VRET can be effective in treating trauma if one is able tolerate these approaches. The avoidance of such approaches is what fuels the need for alternative methods.

Transcranial Magnetic Stimulation

Transcranial magnetic stimulation (TMS) creates a magnetic field by sending a variable current through a coil that induces a firing of selected neuronal areas in the brain. TMS has been used for treatment of depression, reportedly with some success. Although depression is a major component of PTSD, to date, scant empirical evidence from well-controlled studies shows that TMS is a treatment of choice for PTSD itself. TMS is costly and labor-intensive and is in its infancy in terms of its utility in treating trauma. It lacks a consistent body of empirical support for treatment of PTSD.

Internet- and Computer-Based Treatments and Teletherapy

A number of computer-based approaches to treating PTSD exist and go by names such as "Interapy," "guided Internet CBT for PTSD," "Calm," "PTSD Online," "DE-STRESS," "VetChange," and "Vets Prevail." For younger, computer-literate individuals, computer-based approaches do have some allure, and they are also accessible to anyone else with basic computer skills. However, these approaches seem to be comparatively lacking in compelling empirical support, and, oddly, they appear to have a dropout rate that exceeds most other forms of treatment for PTSD. It is unclear why the dropout rate is so high, but it may be that one needs a high level of motivation and self-discipline to push themselves to deliberately stay with these programs, especially when they have to deal with traumatic experiences.

Teletherapy, in which one communicates with a therapist via communication tools, such as Skype or Zoom, may address these dropout issues, but this form of therapy for PTSD typically uses CBT and exposure approaches, and, as a result, may itself result in high dropout. The evidence for the efficacy of tele-therapy in treating PTSD is scant.

Overall, computer-based therapies lack an abundance of evidence support-ing them, but to be fair, there is no substantial evidence that they are not viable as general psychotherapy approaches. Teletherapy is clearly of value for those that have difficulty attending face-to-face therapy sessions, but whether it or computer-based approaches are of value in treating PTSD are unanswered questions.

Neurofeedback

Neurofeedback provides information on the brain's activity and allows those receiving this information to alter the activity by using relaxation, focusing, mental imagery, and meditative procedures. Van der Kolk (2014) reported that those with PTSD often show abnormal and erratic activity in the tempo-ral lobes, and that neurofeedback can help normalize these brain patterns and thereby increase emotional stability (p. 321). Although a number of convinc-ing reports indicate that neurofeedback can increase mental clarity, improve concentration, and produce a calm mental state, few compelling studies show it to be an effective treatment for PTSD. Over the years, approximately 3,000 neurofeedback studies have been conducted, but only a handful have used double blind procedures with sham feedback controls—and they do not provide compelling data supporting the beneficial impact of neurofeedback for PTSD treatment beyond placebo effects (Thibault & Raz, 2017).

Propranolol Therapy

Propranolol is a noradrenergic beta-receptor blocker (beta blocker) that was developed in the 1960s and has been used for decades to treat high blood pressure, angina, and arrhythmias. More recently, propranolol has been used to reduce the impact of phobias and the intense fears associated with PTSD. Rather than erase trauma memories, propranolol works to separate the intense emotional response associated with these memories. In a 2018 study, Brunet et al. conducted a double blind, placebo-controlled, randomized clinical trial with adults suffering from PTSD. Propranolol was administered 90 minutes before a brief trauma memory reactivation session once a week for 6 weeks. Overall results showed significant reductions on psychometrically valid and reliable measures of PTSD in comparison with placebo controls. Replication studies involving long-term follow-ups are clearly needed, but propranolol therapy shows promise as an alternative therapy for PTSD—or, at the very least, as a means of reducing the emotional reactivity associated with this disorder.

Stellate Ganglion Block

Similar to propranolol therapy, *stellate ganglion block* (SGB) is a novel approach to reducing PTSD symptoms that again does not have a solid empirical foundation but has aroused recent interest and funding from the U.S. Department of Defense. SGBs are procedures that involve injection of a local anesthetic into the sympathetic nerves found in the neck area. The procedure has been used primarily for the alleviation of pain, such as severe headaches, refractory angina, and complex regional pain in the upper extremities. It also has been used for arterial vascular insufficiency disorders, such as seen in Reynaud's disease, vasospasm, and arterial embolism. Although SGB does not have a solid research foundation, such as double blind, random controlled investigations for treating PTSD, studies are being done that show promising results. For example, Lynch et al. (2016) used the procedure with 30 active military combat veterans who had multiple deployments and who suffered from PTSD. Overall results showed greatest improvements on a military PTSD symptom checklist in the first week after SGB for irritability, concentration problems, angry outbursts, and sleep problems. After 2 to 4 months, improvements were seen in the areas of feeling distant, cut off, and remote, and, importantly, the authors found a significant reduction in hyperarousal and avoidance symptoms. The reduction in avoidance symptoms is of real importance because avoidance is one of the major reasons why people with PTSD avoid traditional treatments. Long-term follow-up and replication studies are needed.

The Department of Defense has shown an interest in SGB simply because traditional pharmacological and psychological therapies for PTSD are often ineffective or avoided altogether, and the costs for treating PTSD are hugely burdensome. It is likely that efforts will continue to help reduce treatment costs and ongoing work will seek alternative and effective treatments for PTSD.

MY PERSONAL USE OF ALTERNATIVE APPROACHES

At the outset of this book, I mentioned that I had personally experienced trauma by way of the war in Vietnam, where I served in the U.S. Army. The thought of going to the VHA and seeking treatment has caused such a level of anxiety and extreme discomfort that I've avoided doing so for almost 50 years. Half a century of avoidance can give the reader an idea of how big a problem avoidance really is. I have only recently made some visits to the VHA and have found those visits to be highly disturbing despite the kindness exhibited by VHA personnel. I am trying, though, to confront my fears by persisting to visit. I have actually used many of the approaches to treating PTSD that I have described in this book.

I do mindfulness meditation every day, usually in the mornings, for at least 20 minutes. During these sessions, I attempt to maintain a focus on my breathing, body sensations, and mental and emotional preoccupations. I observe and note mental and emotional preoccupations but make every effort to not wade in them and pursue them. In mindfulness meditation, one views their issues almost as an outsider might view another person's concerns. This perspective helps avoid becoming carried away by one's issues and difficulties, including trauma-related ones, but rather to put those issues and difficulties into perspective.

I also pursue AAT, NAT, and exercise with daily jogs through a local arboretum, accompanied by my toy poodle, Sofie. These daily experiences are deeply calming. I also practice yoga at least once a week. Having been trained in EMDR, I also have sat as the client in a few sessions of this procedure and found it to be surprisingly helpful. So, I have taken the alternative "medicine" that has been "prescribed" in this book by engaging in the majority of approaches I have written about.

FINAL NOTE TO CLINICIANS

Those who regularly treat psychological trauma reactions and PTSD have doubtlessly experienced the frustration of trying to help these troubled individuals only to have them quit therapy because the process of confronting their problems is simply too overwhelming to consider. Traditional CBT and PE are highly valuable psychotherapeutic tools that clinicians can use to treat a wide range of psychological problems. However, when these problems involve the extreme levels of anxiety that are precipitated by traumatic experiences, the traditional approaches simply come up short. I hope that the alternative approaches I have presented here can serve as tools that clinicians might consider using with treatment-resistant and treatment-avoidant cases. An additional benefit of the alternative approaches is that they can serve as gateways to traditional treatment. The traumatized individual might be more amenable to trying CBT if they have first eased into dealing with their trauma through yoga, meditation, exercise, and similar alternative approaches.

The goal for clinicians is always client betterment. If alternative approaches are the means to achieving that goal, it is alternative approaches that each clinician should seriously consider. I hope that the alternatives presented in this book will serve the goal of alleviating the suffering of those carrying the weight of PTSD.

Resources for Trauma Sufferers and Clinicians

Much of the material on the various alternative treatments for posttraumatic stress disorder (PTSD) describes the techniques and summarizes the relevant research. Additional textual and video material is provided in this Appendix. This information is presented to enhance understanding of the alternative approaches and, in many instances, to show how the techniques are applied in practice.

EYE-MOVEMENT DESENSITIZATION AND REPROCESSING

Publications

Luber, M. (2009). *Eye movement desensitization and reprocessing (EMDR) scripted protocols: Basics and special situations.* New York, NY: Springer.

Marich, J. (2011). *EMDR made simple: 4 approaches to using EMDR with every client.* Eau Claire, WI: Premier Publishing & Media.

Parnell, L. (2007). *A therapist's guide to EMDR: Tools and techniques for successful treatment.* New York, NY: Norton.

Shapiro, F. (2001). *Eye movement desensitization and reprocessing: Basic principles, protocols and procedures* (2nd ed.). New York, NY: Guilford Press.

Shapiro, F. (2012). *Getting past your past: Take control of your life with self-help techniques from EMDR therapy.* Emmaus, PA: Rodale.

van der Kolk, B. A., Levine, P. A., Parnell, L., & Grand, D. (2015). *EMDR step-by-step: In session demonstrations.* Eau Claire, WI: Pesi.

Internet and Video

Eye Movement Desensitization and Reprocessing (EMDR) Procedure: https://youtu.be/gZ5MLn1Cc94

EMDR Demonstration Phases 1–8: https://youtu.be/L6UvKhLYf7w

Use of EMDR to Get Over a Breakup: https://youtu.be/KpRQvcW2kUM

EMDR's Relevancy to Victims of Child Abuse and Domestic Violence: https://binged.it/2Jxn7Ah

EMDR for Children: https://youtu.be/NEpeGqNz1mA

YOGA

Publications

Cope, S. (1999). *Yoga and the quest for the true self.* New York, NY: Bantam Books.

Emerson, D., & Hopper, E. (2011). *Overcoming trauma through yoga: Reclaiming your body.* Berkeley, CA: North Atlantic Books.

Iyengar, B. K. S. (1966). *Light on yoga.* New York, NY: Schocken Books.

Levine, P. (2010). *In an unspoken voice: How the body releases trauma and restores goodness.* Berkeley, CA: North Atlantic Books.

Miller, R. C. (2015). *The iRest program for healing PTSD: A proven-effective approach to using yoga nidra meditation & deep relaxation techniques to overcome trauma.* Oakland, CA: New Harbinger.

van der Kolk, B. A. (2014). *The body keeps the score: Brain, mind, and body in the healing of trauma.* New York, NY: Viking.

Internet and Video

Yoga for Posttraumatic Stress Disorder: https://youtu.be/TqVSwY8y3UY

Yoga for Overcoming Trauma—With Bessell van der Kolk: https://youtu.be/MmKfzbHzm_s

Three-Part Yoga Breath to Reduce Anxiety From Complex PTSD: https://youtu.be/BcMAfywIFR8

Yoga for After a Disaster: https://www.youtube.com/watch?v=hs73lvN0l8A

Yoga Class for Stress and Trauma—With Five Parks Yoga: https://www.youtube.com/watch?v=oWZ_VQXT4vg

MEDITATION

Publications

Davis, L. (2017). *Meditations for healing trauma: Mindfulness skills to ease post-traumatic stress.* Oakland, CA: New Harbinger.

Germer, C. K., Siegel, R. D., & Fulton, P. R. (2005). *Mindfulness and psychotherapy.* New York, NY: Guilford Press.

Kabat-Zinn, J. (1994). *Wherever you go, there you are: Mindfulness meditations in everyday life.* New York, NY: Hyperion.

Kabat-Zinn, J. (2005). *Coming to our senses: Healing ourselves and the world through mindfulness.* New York, NY: Hyperion.

Kabat-Zinn, J. (2013). *Full catastrophe living: Using the wisdom of your body and mind to face stress, pain, and illness.* New York, NY: Bantam Books.

Kornfield, J. (2009). *A path with heart: A guide through the perils and promises of spiritual life.* New York, NY: Bantam Books.

Tarrant, J. (2017). *Meditation interventions to rewire the brain: Integrating neuroscience strategies for ADHD, anxiety, depression and PTSD.* Eau Claire, WI: Pesi.

Turow, R. G. (2017). *Mindfulness skills for trauma and PTSD.* New York, NY: Norton.

Internet and Video

PTSD Visualization for Trauma Relief and Healing: https://www.youtube.com/watch?v=H8e4sATalz8

Mindfulness Meditations for Releasing Trauma: https://www.youtube.com/watch?v=AvqMP8tI6bw

Guided Meditation for Complex PTSD: https://www.youtube.com/watch?v=RahidNEDtt0

Guided Meditation for Complex PTSD That Focuses on Healing and Wholeness: https://www.youtube.com/watch?v=IpEMQ0Xq1sk

Guided Meditation for PTSD: https://www.youtube.com/watch?v=bFBulCQ0u0k

Power of Meditation to Overcome Traumatic Experiences: A PTSD Case Study: https://www.youtube.com/watch?v=MxnDRP_0J58

EXERCISE, TRAUMA, AND NEGATIVE EMOTIONAL STATES

Publications

de Moor, M. H. M., Beem, A. L., Stubbe, J. H., Boomsma, D. I., & De Geus, E. J. C. (2006). Regular exercise, anxiety, depression and personality: A population-based study. *Preventive Medicine, 42,* 273–279. http://dx.doi.org/10.1016/j.ypmed.2005.12.002

Hays, K. F. (1999). *Working it out: Using exercise in psychotherapy.* Washington, DC: American Psychological Association. http://dx.doi.org/10.1037/10333-000

Manger, T. A., & Motta, R. W. (2005). The impact of an exercise program on posttraumatic stress disorder, anxiety, and depression. *International Journal of Emergency Mental Health, 7,* 49–57.

Motta, R. W. (2018, Summer). The role of exercise in alleviating anxiety, depression, and PTSD. *Behavioral Health News,* pp. 33, 37. Retrieved from http://mhnews.org/back_issues/BHN-Summer2018.pdf

Motta, R. W. (2018). The role of exercise in reducing PTSD and negative emotional states. In S. G. Taukeni (Ed.), *Psychology of health—Biopsychosocial approach.* http://dx.doi.org/10.5772/intechopen.81012. Retrieved from https://www.intechopen.com/books/psychology-of-health-biopsychosocial-approach/the-role-of-exercise-in-reducing-ptsd-and-negative-emotional-states

Motta, R. W., McWilliams, M. E., Schwartz, J. T., & Cavera, R. S. (2012). The role of exercise in reducing childhood and adolescent PTSD, anxiety, and depression. *Journal of Applied School Psychology, 28,* 224–238. http://dx.doi.org/10.1080/15377903.2012.695765

Shivakumar, G., Anderson, E. H., Surís, A. M., & North, C. S. (2017). Exercise for PTSD in women veterans: A proof-of-concept study. *Military Medicine, 182,* e1809–e1814. http://dx.doi.org/10.7205/MILMED-D-16-00440

Whitworth, J. W., Craft, L. L., Dunsiger, S. I., & Ciccolo, J. T. (2017). Direct and indirect effects of exercise on posttraumatic stress disorder symptoms: A longitudinal study. *General Hospital Psychiatry, 49,* 56–62. http://dx.doi.org/10.1016/j.genhosppsych.2017.06.012

Internet and Video

Relief of PTSD Symptoms Through Exercise: https://youtu.be/iIOquRSeBos
Exercise Management for Depression: https://youtu.be/ILRqYb4ZPrk
Exercise to Heal Trauma: https://youtu.be/CZVH4J6Kk_Q

NATURE- AND ANIMAL-ASSISTED THERAPIES

Publications

Annerstedt, M., & Währborg, P. (2011). Nature-assisted therapy: Systematic review of controlled and observational studies. *Scandinavian Journal of Public Health, 39,* 371–388. http://dx.doi.org/10.1177/1403494810396400

Gabrielsen, L. E., Fernee, C. R., Aasen, G. O., & Eskedal, L. T. (2016). Why randomized trials are challenging within adventure therapy research: Lessons learned in Norway. *Journal of Experiential Education, 39,* 5–14. http://dx.doi.org/10.1177/1053825915607535

Neill, J. T. (2003). Reviewing and benchmarking adventure therapy outcomes: Applications of meta-analysis. *Journal of Experiential Education, 25,* 316–321. http://dx.doi.org/10.1177/105382590302500305

O'Haire, M. E., & Rodriguez, K. E. (2018). Preliminary efficacy of service dogs as a complementary treatment for posttraumatic stress disorder in military members and veterans. *Journal of Consulting and Clinical Psychology, 86,* 179–188. http://dx.doi.org/10.1037/ccp0000267

Relf, P. D. (2005). The therapeutic values of plants. *Pediatric Rehabilitation, 8,* 235–237. http://dx.doi.org/10.1080/13638490400011140

Williams, F. (2017). *The nature fix.* New York, NY: Norton.

Yarborough, B. J. H., Stumbo, S. P., Yarborough, M. T., Owen-Smith, A., & Green, C. A. (2018). Benefits and challenges of using service dogs for veterans with posttraumatic stress disorder. *Psychiatric Rehabilitation Journal, 41,* 118–124. http://dx.doi.org/10.1037/prj0000294

Internet and Video

Web Article on Animals and Emotional Health: https://www.uclahealth.org/pac/animal-assisted-therapy
Adventure Therapy for PTSD: https://youtu.be/YM9wPT2geYs
Dogs Helping to Facilitate Recovery From Medical Procedures: https://youtu.be/XNqvC9cWhuE
Horses as a Therapeutic Adjunct for PTSD: https://youtu.be/Z7EedCwJ4ww

ACUPUNCTURE FOR TRAUMA AND PTSD

Publications

Abbate, S. (2018). *Acupuncture strategies for complex patients: From consultation to treatment.* Philadelphia, PA: Singing Dragon.

Gash, M. R., & Henning, B. A. (2004). *Acupressure for emotional healing: A self-care guide for trauma, stress, & common emotional imbalances.* New York, NY: Bantam Dell.

Hollifield, M. (2011). Acupuncture for posttraumatic stress disorder: Conceptual, clinical, and biological data support further research. *CNS Neuroscience & Therapeutics, 17,* 769–779. http://dx.doi.org/10.1111/j.1755-5949.2011.00241.x

Hollifield, M., Sinclair-Lian, N., Warner, T. D., & Hammerschlag, R. (2007). Acupuncture for posttraumatic stress disorder: A randomized controlled pilot trial. *Journal of Nervous and Mental Disease, 195,* 504–513. http://dx.doi.org/10.1097/NMD.0b013e31803044f8

Holman, C. T. (2017). *Treating emotional trauma with Chinese medicine: Integrated diagnostic and treatment strategies.* Philadelphia, PA: Singing Dragon.

Internet and Video

Web Article on Acupuncture for Military PTSD Service Personnel: https://www.healthcmi.com/Acupuncture-Continuing-Education-News/1410-acupuncture-for-combat-ptsd-found-effective
Acupuncture for Anxiety and PTSD: https://youtu.be/BZ7guRWiurE

Acupuncture for PTSD: https://youtu.be/eEgzCnBS1vo
Navy Veteran Treated for PTSD With Acupuncture: https://youtu.be/iIlqG9gRU2k

EMOTIONAL FREEDOM TECHNIQUES

Publications

Craig, G. (2008). *EFT for PTSD*. Fulton, CA: Energy Psychology Press.

Dhond, R. P., Kettner, N., & Napadow, V. (2007). Neuroimaging acupuncture effects in the human brain. *Journal of Alternative and Complementary Medicine, 13*, 603–616. http://dx.doi.org/10.1089/acm.2007.7040

Ortner, N. (2013). *The tapping solution: A revolutionary system for stress-free living*. New York, NY: Hay House.

Ortner, N. (2015). *The tapping solution for pain relief: A step-by-step guide to reducing and eliminating chronic pain*. New York, NY: Hay House.

Sebastian, B., & Nelms, J. (2017). The effectiveness of emotional freedom techniques in the treatment of posttraumatic stress disorder: A meta-analysis. *Explore, 13*, 16–25. http://dx.doi.org/10.1016/j.explore.2016.10.001

Varvogli, L., & Darviri, C. (2011). Stress management techniques: Evidence-based procedures that reduce stress and promote health. *Health Science Journal, 5*, 74–89.

Internet and Video

Emotional Freedom Techniques (EFT) and Basic Self-Care: https://youtu.be/TRq8o1MEUtU

EFT for Troubling Aspects of Life: https://youtu.be/IWu3rSEddZI

EFT for Trauma and Abuse: https://youtu.be/vcWlBld1SqU

EFT for PTSD: https://youtu.be/gJm5b3Y-Vug

EFT and Childhood Trauma: https://youtu.be/T-4c-9HzsO8

MDMA—ECSTASY

Publications

Mithoefer, M. C. (2017). *A manual for MDMA-assisted psychotherapy in the treatment of posttraumatic stress disorder* (Version 8.1). Santa Cruz, CA: Multidisciplinary Association for Psychedelic Studies. Retrieved from https://s3-us-west-1.amazonaws.com/mapscontent/research-archive/mdma/TreatmentManual_MDMAAssistedPsychotherapyVersion+8.1_22+Aug2017.pdf

Mithoefer, M. C., Wagner, M. T., Mithoefer, A. T., Jerome, L., & Doblin, R. (2011). The safety and efficacy of ±3,4-methylenedioxymethamphetamine-assisted psychotherapy in subjects with chronic, treatment-resistant posttraumatic stress disorder: The first randomized controlled pilot study. *Journal of Psychopharmacology, 25*, 439–452. http://dx.doi.org/10.1177/0269881110378371

Oehen, P., Traber, R., Widmer, V., & Schnyder, U. (2013). A randomized, controlled pilot study of MDMA (3,4-methylenedioxymethamphetamine)-assisted psychotherapy for treatment of resistant, chronic post-traumatic stress disorder (PTSD). *Journal of Psychopharmacology, 27*, 40–52. http://dx.doi.org/10.1177/0269881112464827

Other, A. (2017). *Trust, surrender, receive: How MDMA can release us from trauma and PTSD*. Carson City, NV: Lioncrest.

Sessa, B. (2017). MDMA and PTSD treatment: "PTSD: From novel pathophysiology to innovative therapeutics." *Neuroscience Letters, 649*, 176–180. http://dx.doi.org/10.1016/j.neulet.2016.07.004

Internet and Video

Web Article on 3,4-Methylenedioxymethamphetamine, or MDMA ("Ecstasy"), Including History and Side Effects: https://www.thoughtco.com/invention-of-mdma-ecstasy-4079861

Web Article "Ecstasy as a Remedy for PTSD? You Probably Have Some Questions" in *The New York Times:* https://www.nytimes.com/2018/05/01/us/ecstasy-molly-ptsd-mdma.html

Army Veteran's Story About MDMA Use for PTSD: https://youtu.be/8K5sJuTbQvY

MDMA for PTSD: A Case Study: https://youtu.be/O3DAI_n-PO4

Ted Talk on MDMA and Trauma: https://youtu.be/KPMp7xEvcXk

REFERENCES

Abdill, M. N., & Juppé, D. (2005). *Pets in therapy: Animal assisted activities in health care facilities.* Ravensdale, WA: Idyll Arbor.

Alfermann, D., & Stoll, O. (Eds.). (2005). *Sportpsychologie: Ein Lehrbuch in 12 Lektionen* [Sports psychology: A textbook in 12 lessons]. Aachen, Germany: Meyer & Meyer Verlag.

Altchiler, L., & Motta, R. (1994). Effects of aerobic and nonaerobic exercise on anxiety, absenteeism, and job satisfaction. *Journal of Clinical Psychology, 50,* 829–840. http://dx.doi.org/10.1002/1097-4679(199411)50:6%3C829::AID-JCLP2270500603%3E3.0.CO;2-I

Alvarez, J., McLean, C., Harris, A. H., Rosen, C. S., Ruzek, J. I., & Kimerling, R. (2011). The comparative effectiveness of cognitive processing therapy for male veterans treated in a VHA posttraumatic stress disorder residential rehabilitation program. *Journal of Consulting and Clinical Psychology, 79,* 590–599. http://dx.doi.org/10.1037/a0024466

American Psychiatric Association. (1980). *Diagnostic and statistical manual of mental disorders* (3rd ed.). Washington, DC: Author.

American Psychiatric Association. (1994). *Diagnostic and statistical manual of mental disorders* (4th ed.). Washington, DC: Author.

American Psychiatric Association. (2013). *Diagnostic and statistical manual of mental disorders* (5th ed.). Washington, DC: Author.

Ames, D., & Wirshing, W. C. (1993). Ecstasy, the serotonin syndrome, and neuroleptic malignant syndrome—A possible link? *JAMA, 269,* 869–870. http://dx.doi.org/10.1001/jama.1993.03500070049022

Amstadter, A. B., & Vernon, L. L. (2008). Emotional reactions during and after trauma: A comparison of trauma types. *Journal of Aggression, Maltreatment & Trauma, 16,* 391–408. http://dx.doi.org/10.1080/10926770801926492

Annerstedt, M., & Währborg, P. (2011). Nature-assisted therapy: Systematic review of controlled and observational studies. *Scandinavian Journal of Public Health, 39,* 371–388. http://dx.doi.org/10.1177/1403494810396400

Annesi, J. J. (2004). Relationship between self-efficacy and changes in rated tension and depression for 9- to 12-yr.-old children enrolled in a 12-wk. after-school physical activity program. *Perceptual and Motor Skills, 99,* 191–194. http://dx.doi.org/10.2466/PMS.99.5.191-194

Annesi, J. J. (2005). Improvements in self-concept associated with reductions in negative mood in preadolescents enrolled in an after-school physical activity program. *Psychological Reports, 97,* 400–404. http://dx.doi.org/10.2466/PR0.97.6.400-404

APA Presidential Task Force on Evidence-Based Practice. (2006). Evidence-based practice in psychology. *American Psychologist, 61,* 271–285. Retrieved from https://psycnet.apa.org/fulltext/2006-05893-001.html

Assefi, N. P., Sherman, K. J., Jacobsen, C., Goldberg, J., Smith, W. R., & Buchwald, D. (2005). A randomized clinical trial of acupuncture compared with sham acupuncture in fibromyalgia. *Annals of Internal Medicine, 143,* 10–19. http://dx.doi.org/10.7326/0003-4819-143-1-200507050-00005

Bakker, G. M. (2013). The current status of energy psychology: Extraordinary claims with less than ordinary evidence. *Clinical Psychologist, 17,* 91–99. http://dx.doi.org/10.1111/cp.12020

Bandura, A. (1997). *Self-efficacy: The exercise of control.* New York, NY: Freeman.

Banks, K., Newman, E., & Saleem, J. (2015). An overview of the research on mindfulness-based interventions for treating symptoms of posttraumatic stress disorder: A systematic review. *Journal of Clinical Psychology, 71,* 935–963. http://dx.doi.org/10.1002/jclp.22200

Barrowcliff, A. L., Gray, N. S., MacCulloch, S., Freeman, T. C. A., & MacCulloch, M. J. (2003). Horizontal rhythmical eye movements consistently diminish the arousal provoked by auditory stimuli. *British Journal of Clinical Psychology, 42,* 289–302. http://dx.doi.org/10.1348/01446650360703393

Beck, M. (2010, December 21). Beside Freud's couch, a chow named Jofi. *The Wall Street Journal.* Retrieved from https://www.wsj.com/articles/SB10001424052748703886904576031630124087362

Bender, B. B. (2014). *Yoga for warriors: Basic training in strength, resilience, and peace of mind—A system for veterans & military service men and women.* Boulder, CO: Sounds True.

Benson, H. (1975). *The relaxation response.* New York, NY: Morrow.

Berk, M. (2007). Should we be targeting exercise as a routine mental health intervention? *Acta Neuropsychiatrica, 19,* 217–218. http://dx.doi.org/10.1111/j.1601-5215.2007.00201.x

Berman, B. M., Lao, L., Langenberg, P., Lee, W. L., Gilpin, A. M. K., & Hochberg, M. C. (2004). Effectiveness of acupuncture as adjunctive therapy in osteoarthritis of the knee: A randomized, controlled trial. *Annals of Internal Medicine, 141,* 901–910. http://dx.doi.org/10.7326/0003-4819-141-12-200412210-00006

Bernschneider-Reif, S., Oxler, F., & Freudenmann, R. W. (2006). The origin of MDMA ("Ecstasy"): Separating the facts from the myth. *Die Pharmazie, 61,* 966–972.

Biophilia hypothesis. (n.d.). In *Wikipedia.* Retrieved from https://en.wikipedia.org/wiki/Biophilia_hypothesis

Blake, D. D., Weathers, F., Nagy, L. M., Kaloupek, D. G., Klauminzer, G., Charney, D. S., & Keane, T. M. (1990). A clinician rating scale for assessing current and lifetime PTSD: The CAPS-1. *Behavior Therapist, 13*, 187–188.

Blanchard, E. B., Hickling, E. J., Buckley, T. C., Taylor, A. E., Vollmer, A., & Loos, W. R. (1996). Psychophysiology of posttraumatic stress disorder related to motor vehicle accidents: Replication and extension. *Journal of Consulting and Clinical Psychology, 64*, 742–751. http://dx.doi.org/10.1037/0022-006X.64.4.742

Boccio, F. J. (2004). *Mindfulness yoga: The awakened union of breath, body and mind.* Boston, MA: Wisdom.

Bodin, T., & Martinsen, E. W. (2004). Mood and self-efficacy during acute exercise in clinical depression: A randomized, controlled study. *Journal of Sport and Exercise Psychology, 26*, 623–633. http://dx.doi.org/10.1123/jsep.26.4.623

Boscarino, J. A., Adams, R. E., Figley, C. R., Galea, S., & Foa, E. B. (2006). Fear of terrorism and preparedness in New York City 2 years after the attacks: Implications for disaster planning and research. *Journal of Public Health Management and Practice, 12*, 505–513.

Bougea, A. M., Spandideas, N., Alexopoulos, E. C., Thomaides, T., Chrousos, G. P., & Darviri, C. (2013). Effect of the emotional freedom technique on perceived stress, quality of life, and cortisol salivary levels in tension-type headache sufferers: A randomized controlled trial. *Explore, 9*, 91–99. http://dx.doi.org/10.1016/j.explore.2012.12.005

Bowen, D. J., & Neill, J. T. (2013). A meta-analysis of adventure therapy outcomes and moderators. *Open Psychology Journal, 6*, 28–53. http://dx.doi.org/10.2174/1874350120130802001

Bradley, R., Greene, J., Russ, E., Dutra, L., & Westen, D. (2005). A multidimensional meta-analysis of psychotherapy for PTSD. *American Journal of Psychiatry, 162*, 214–227. http://dx.doi.org/10.1176/appi.ajp.162.2.214

Bravo, G. L. (2001). What does MDMA feel like? In J. Holland (Ed.), *Ecstasy: The complete guide—A comprehensive look at the risks and benefits of MDMA* (pp. 21–28). Rochester, VT: Park Street Press.

Breslau, N. (2009). The epidemiology of trauma, PTSD, and other posttrauma disorders. *Trauma, Violence, & Abuse, 10*, 198–210. http://dx.doi.org/10.1177/1524838009334448

A brief organizational history. (n.d.). Retrieved from https://hanuman-foundation.org/about.html

Brumbaugh, A. G. (1993). Acupuncture: New perspective in chemical dependency treatment. *Journal of Substance Abuse Treatment, 10*, 35–43. http://dx.doi.org/10.1016/0740-5472(93)90096-K

Brunet, A., Saumier, D., Liu, A., Streiner, D. L., Tremblay, J., & Pitman, R. K. (2018). Reduction of PTSD symptoms with pre-activation propranolol therapy: A randomized controlled trial. *American Journal of Psychiatry, 175*, 427–433. http://dx.doi.org/10.1176/appi.ajp.2017.17050481

Bryant, R. A., Moulds, M. I., Mastrodomenico, J., Hopwood, S., Felmingham, K., & Nixon, R. D. V. (2007). Who drops out of treatment for post-traumatic stress disorder? *Clinical Psychologist, 11*, 13–15. http://dx.doi.org/10.1080/13284200601178128

Bushman, B. (Ed.). (2017). *ACSM's complete guide to fitness & health* (2nd ed.). Champaign, IL: Human Kinetics.

Buzel, A. H. (2016). *Beyond words: The healing power of horses—Bridging the worlds of equine assisted therapy and psychotherapy.* Bloomington, IN: AuthorHouse.

Callahan, R. (1997). Thought field therapy: The case of Mary. *Traumatology, 3,* 30–37. http://dx.doi.org/10.1177/153476569700300105

Callahan, R. J., & Callahan, J. (2000). *Stop the nightmares of trauma.* Chapel Hill, NC: Professional Press.

Carlson, J. G., Chemtob, C. M., Rusnak, K., Hedlund, N. L., & Muraoka, M. Y. (1998). Eye movement desensitization and reprocessing (EDMR) treatment for combat-related posttraumatic stress disorder. *Journal of Traumatic Stress, 11,* 3–24. http://dx.doi.org/10.1023/A:1024448814268

Center for Deployment Psychology. (n.d.). Prolonged exposure therapy for PTSD (PE). Retrieved from https://deploymentpsych.org/treatments/prolonged-exposure-therapy-ptsd-pe

Center for Mindfulness in Medicine, Health Care, and Society. (n.d.). History of MBSR. Retrieved from https://www.umassmed.edu/cfm/mindfulness-based-programs/mbsr-courses/about-mbsr/history-of-mbsr/

Chemtob, C. M., Tolin, D. F., van der Kolk, B. A., & Pitman, R. K. (2000). Eye movement desensitization and reprocessing. In E. B. Foa, T. M. Keane, & M. J. Friedman (Eds.), *Effective treatments for PTSD: Practice guidelines from the International Society for Traumatic Stress Studies* (pp. 139–154). New York, NY: Guilford Press.

Church, D. (2013). Clinical EFT as an evidence-based practice for the treatment of psychological and physiological conditions. *Psychology, 4,* 645–654. http://dx.doi.org/10.4236/psych.2013.48092

Church, D., & Feinstein, D. (2013). Energy psychology in the treatment of PTSD: Psychobiology and clinical principles. In T. Van Leeuwen & M. Brouwer (Eds.), *Psychology of trauma* (pp. 211–224). Hauppage, NY: Nova Science.

Church, D., Feinstein, D., Palmer-Hoffman, J. Stein, P. K., & Tranguch, A. (2014). Empirically supported psychological treatments: The challenge of evaluating clinical innovations. *Journal of Nervous and Mental Disease, 202,* 699–709. http://dx.doi.org/10.1097/NMD.0000000000000188

Church, D., Hawk, C., Brooks, A. J., Toukolehto, O., Wren, M., Dinter, I., & Stein, P. (2013). Psychological trauma symptom improvement in veterans using emotional freedom techniques: A randomized controlled trial. *Journal of Nervous and Mental Disease, 201,* 153–160. http://dx.doi.org/10.1097/NMD.0b013e31827f6351

Church, D., & Nelms, J. (2016). Pain, range of motion, and psychological symptoms in a population with frozen shoulder: A randomized controlled dismantling study of clinical EFT (emotional freedom techniques). *Archives of Scientific Psychology, 4,* 38–48. http://dx.doi.org/10.1037/arc0000028

Church, D., Piña, O., Reategui, C., & Brooks, A. (2012). Single-session reduction of the intensity of traumatic memories in abused adolescents after EFT: A randomized controlled pilot study. *Traumatology, 18,* 73–79. http://dx.doi.org/10.1177/1534765611426788

Church, D., Yount, G., & Brooks, A. J. (2012). The effect of emotional freedom techniques on stress biochemistry: A randomized controlled trial. *Journal of Nervous and Mental Disease, 200,* 891–896. http://dx.doi.org/10.1097/NMD.0b013e31826b9fcl

Cirrik, S., & Hacioglu, G. (2016). *Neurophysiological effects of exercise.* http://dx.doi.org/10.5772/64801

Clark, M. A. (1903). Memoir of J. M. Da Costa, MD. *Journal of the Medical Sciences,* 318–329.

Cloitre, M., Garvert, D. W., Weiss, B., Carlson, E. B., & Bryant, R. A. (2014). Distinguishing PTSD, complex PTSD, and borderline personality disorder: A latent class analysis. *European Journal of Psychotraumatology, 5,* 25097. Advance online publication. http://dx.doi.org/10.3402/ejpt.v5.25097

Cloitre, M., Stolbach, B. C., Herman, J. L., van der Kolk, B., Pynoos, R., Wang, J., & Petkova, E. (2009). A developmental approach to complex PTSD: Childhood and adult cumulative trauma as predictors of symptom complexity. *Journal of Traumatic Stress, 22,* 399–408. http://dx.doi.org/10.1002/jts.20444

Cohen, J. (1987). *Statistical power analysis for the behavioral sciences.* Hillside, NJ: Erlbaum.

Congressional Budget Office. (2012). *The Veterans Health Administration's treatment of PTSD and traumatic brain injury among recent combat veterans* (Pub. No. 4097). Retrieved from https://www.cbo.gov/sites/default/files/112th-congress-2011-2012/reports/02-09-PTSD_0.pdf

Controlled Substances Act, Pub. L. 91-513, title II, Oct. 27, 1970, 84 Stat. 1242 (21 U.S.C. 801 et seq.).

Costello, E. J., Mustillo, S., Erkanli, A., Keeler, G., & Angold, A. (2003). Prevalence and development of psychiatric disorders in childhood and adolescence. *Archives of General Psychiatry, 60,* 837–844. http://dx.doi.org/10.1001/archpsyc.60.8.837

Crews, D. J., Lochbaum, M. R., & Landers, D. M. (2004). Aerobic physical activity effects on psychological well-being in low-income Hispanic children. *Perceptual and Motor Skills, 98,* 319–324. http://dx.doi.org/10.2466/pms.98.1.319-324

Daly, R. J. (1983). Samuel Pepys and post-traumatic stress disorder. *British Journal of Psychiatry, 143,* 64–68. http://dx.doi.org/10.1192/bjp.143.1.64

Damasio, A. (2010). *Self comes to mind: Constructing the conscious brain.* New York, NY: Vintage Books.

Dass, R. (1971). *Be here now.* New York, NY: Crown.

Davidson, P. R., & Parker, K. C. H. (2001). Eye movement desensitization and reprocessing (EMDR): A meta-analysis. *Journal of Consulting and Clinical Psychology, 69,* 305–316. http://dx.doi.org/10.1037/0022-006X.69.2.305

DeBoer, L. B., Powers, M. B., Utschig, A. C., Otto, M. W., & Smits, J. A. (2012). Exploring exercise as an avenue for the treatment of anxiety disorders. *Expert Review of Neurotherapeutics, 12,* 1011–1022. http://dx.doi.org/10.1586/ern.12.73

de Moor, M. H. M., Beem, A. L., Stubbe, J. H., Boomsma, D. I., & De Geus, E. J. C. (2006). Regular exercise, anxiety, depression and personality: A population-based study. *Preventive Medicine, 42,* 273–279. http://dx.doi.org/10.1016/j.ypmed.2005.12.002

Developmental history of energy tapping techniques inc TFT, classic TFT & modern energy tapping. (2014, April 29). Retrieved from The Guild of Energists website https://goe.ac/history_of_tapping.htm

Dhond, R. P., Kettner, N., & Napadow, V. (2007). Neuroimaging acupuncture effects in the human brain. *Journal of Alternative and Complementary Medicine, 13,* 603–616. http://dx.doi.org/10.1089/acm.2007.7040

Dialectical behavior therapy. (n.d.). In *Wikipedia.* Retrieved from https://wiki2.org/en/Dialectical_behavior_therapy

Diaz, A. B., & Motta, R. (2008). The effects of an aerobic exercise program on posttraumatic stress disorder symptom severity in adolescents. *International Journal of Emergency Mental Health, 10,* 49–59.

Dick, A. M., Niles, B. L., Street, A. E., DiMartino, D. M., & Mitchell, K. S. (2014). Examining mechanisms of change in a yoga intervention for women: The influence of mindfulness, psychological flexibility, and emotion regulation on PTSD symptoms. *Journal of Clinical Psychology, 70,* 1170–1182. http://dx.doi.org/10.1002/jclp.22104

Dienstmann, G. (2018). *Practical meditation: A simple step-by-step guide.* New York, NY: DK.

Dietrich, A., & McDaniel, W. F. (2004). Endocannabinoids and exercise. *British Journal of Sports Medicine, 38,* 536–541. http://dx.doi.org/10.1136/bjsm.2004.011718

Ding, Q., & Shen, F. (2015). Effects of acupuncture and moxibustion on electrophysiological characteristics of peripheral nerves in patients with carpal tunnel syndrome. *Journal of Clinical and Experimental Medicine, 14*(4).

Donovan, G. H., Butry, D. T., Michael, Y. L., Prestemon, J. P., Liebhold, A. M., Gatziolis, D., & Mao, M. Y. (2013). The relationship between trees and human health: Evidence from the spread of the emerald ash borer. *American Journal of Preventive Medicine, 44,* 139–145. http://dx.doi.org/10.1016/j.amepre.2012.09.066

Dubner, A. E., & Motta, R. W. (1999). Sexually and physically abused foster care children and posttraumatic stress disorder. *Journal of Consulting and Clinical Psychology, 67,* 367–373. http://dx.doi.org/10.1037/0022-006X.67.3.367

Editors of *Encyclopaedia Britannica.* (n.d.). *Stream of consciousness* [Web article]. Retrieved from https://www.britannica.com/art/stream-of-consciousness

Eggiman, J. (2006). Cognitive-behavioral therapy: A case report—Animal assisted therapy. *Topic in Advance practice Nursing eJournal, 6*(3). Retrieved from https://www.medscape.com/viewarticle/545439

Eisenberg, D. M., Cohen, M. H., Hrbek, A., Grayzel, J., Van Rompay, M. I., & Cooper, R. A. (2002). Credentialing complementary and alternative medical providers. *Annals of Internal Medicine, 137,* 965–973.

Elkington, T. J., Cassar, S., Nelson, A. R., & Levinger, I. (2017). Psychological responses to acute aerobic, resistance, or combined exercise in healthy and overweight individuals: A systematic review. *Clinical Insights: Cardiology, 11,* 1–23. http://dx.doi.org/10.1177/1179546817701725

Ellis, A. (1975). *A new guide to rational living.* North Hollywood, CA: Wilshire.

Ellis, A. (1994). Post-traumatic stress disorder (PTSD): A rational emotive behavioral theory. *Journal of Rational-Emotive and Cognitive-Behavior Therapy, 12,* 3–25. http://dx.doi.org/10.1007/BF02354487

Emerson, D., & Hopper, E. (2011). *Overcoming trauma through yoga: Reclaiming your body.* Berkeley, CA: North Atlantic Books.

Emmons, S. L., & Otto, L. (2005). Acupuncture for overactive bladder: A randomized controlled trial. *Obstetrics & Gynecology, 106,* 138–143. http://dx.doi.org/10.1097/01.AOG.0000163258.57895.ec

Emotional freedom techniques. (n.d.). In *Wikipedia.* Retrieved from https://en.wikipedia.org/wiki/Emotional_Freedom_Techniques

Errington-Evans, N. (2012). Acupuncture for anxiety. *CNS Neuroscience & Therapeutics, 18,* 277–284. http://dx.doi.org/10.1111/j.1755-5949.2011.00254.x

Farrell, P. A., Gates, W. K., Maksud, M. G., & Morgan, W. P. (1982). Increases in plasma beta-endorphin/beta-lipotropin immunoreactivity after treadmill running in humans. *Journal of Applied Physiology, 52,* 1245–1249. http://dx.doi.org/10.1152/jappl.1982.52.5.1245

Fatwa, K. (n.d.). Dialectical behavior therapy—DBT tools. Retrieved from https://vidi24.blogspot.com/2017/11/dialectical-behavior-therapy-dbt-tools.html

Feduccia, A. A., Holland, J., & Mithoefer, M. C. (2018). Progress and promise for the MDMA drug development program. *Psychopharmacology*, *235*, 561–571. http://dx.doi.org/10.1007/s00213-017-4779-2

Field, T., Diego, M., & Sanders, C. E. (2001). Exercise is positively related to adolescents' relationships and academics. *Adolescence, 36*, 105–110.

File: Merck patent for synthesizing methylhydrastinine from MDMA. (1914). In *Wikimedia Commons*. Retrieved from https://commons.wikimedia.org/wiki/File:Merck_patent_for_synthesizing_methylhydrastinine_from_MDMA.pdf

Foa, E. B., Hembree, E. A., & Rothbaum, B. O. (2007). *Prolonged exposure therapy for PTSD: Emotional process of traumatic experiences—Therapist guide*. New York, NY: Oxford University Press. http://dx.doi.org/10.1093/med:psych/9780195308501.001.0001

Foa, E. B., Keane, T. M., & Friedman, M. J. (2000). *Effective treatments for PTSD*. New York, NY: Guilford Press.

Foa, E. B., & Kozak, M. J. (1986). Emotional processing of fear: Exposure to corrective information. *Psychological Bulletin, 99*, 20–35. http://dx.doi.org/10.1037/0033-2909.99.1.20

Fox, L. (2013). Is acupoint tapping an active ingredient or an inert placebo in emotional freedom techniques (EFT)? A randomized controlled dismantling study. *Energy Psychology, 5*, 15–26.

Freud, S. (1961). Civilization and its discontents. In J. Strachey (Ed. & Trans.), *The standard edition of the complete psychological works of Sigmund Freud* (Vol. 21, pp. 64–145). London, England: Hogarth Press. (Original work published 1930)

Gabrielsen, L. E., Fernee, C. R., Aasen, G. O., & Eskedal, L. T. (2016). Why randomized trials are challenging within adventure therapy research. *Journal of Experiential Education, 39*, 5–14. http://dx.doi.org/10.1177/1053825915607535

Gaesser, A. H., & Karan, O. C. (2017). A randomized controlled comparison of emotional freedom technique and cognitive-behavioral therapy to reduce adolescent anxiety: A pilot study. *Journal of Alternative and Complementary Medicine, 23*, 102–108. http://dx.doi.org/10.1089/acm.2015.0316

Gallegos, A. M., Crean, H. F., Pigeon, W. R., & Heffner, K. L. (2017). Meditation and yoga for posttraumatic stress disorder: A meta-analytic review of randomized controlled trials. *Clinical Psychology Review, 58*, 115–124. http://dx.doi.org/10.1016/j.cpr.2017.10.004

Garcia, H. A., Kelley, L. P., Rentz, T. O., & Lee, S. (2011). Pretreatment predictors of dropout from cognitive behavioral therapy for PTSD in Iraq and Afghanistan War veterans. *Psychological Services, 8*, 1–11. http://dx.doi.org/10.1037/a0022705

Gaudiano, B. A., Brown, L. A., & Miller, L. W. (2012). Tapping their patients' problems away? Characteristics of psychotherapists using energy meridian techniques. *Research on Social Work Practice, 22*, 647–655. http://dx.doi.org/10.1177/1049731512448468

Germer, C. K. (2005). Mindfulness. What is it? What does it matter? In C. Germer, R. Siegel, & R. Fulton (Eds.), *Mindfulness and psychotherapy* (pp. 3–27). New York, NY: Guilford Press.

Germer, C. K., Siegel, R. D., & Fulton, P. R. (Eds.). (2013). *Mindfulness and psychotherapy* (2nd ed.). New York, NY: Guilford Press.

Ginsburgh, Y. (2006). *What you need to know about Kabbalah*. Kfar Jerusalem, Israel: Gal Einai.

Goodwin, R. D. (2006). Association between coping with anger and feelings of depression among youths. *American Journal of Public Health, 96*, 664–669. http://dx.doi.org/10.2105/AJPH.2004.049742

Gunaratana, B. (2002). *Mindfulness in plain English.* Somerville, MA: Wisdom.

Hamilton, M. (1960). A rating scale for depression. *Journal of Neurology, Neurosurgery and Psychiatry, 23,* 56–62.

Harper, M. (2012). Taming the amygdala: An EEG analysis of exposure therapy for the traumatized. *Traumatology, 18,* 61–74. http://dx.doi.org/10.1177/1534765611429082

Harris, D., & Warren, J. (with Adler, C.). (2017). *Meditation for fidgety skeptics: A 10% happier how-to book.* New York, NY: Spiegel & Grau.

Hartmann, S. (2003). *Adventures in EFT: Your essential guide to emotional freedom* (6th ed.). Eastbourne, England: DragonRising.com.

Hayes, S. C., Follette, V. M., & Linehan, M. N. (Eds.). (2004). *Mindfulness and acceptance: Expanding the cognitive-behavioral tradition.* New York, NY: Guilford Press.

Hayes, S. C., Strosahl, K. D., & Wilson, G. (2016). *Acceptance and commitment therapy: The process and practice of mindful change* (2nd ed.). New York, NY: Guilford Press.

He, G.-h., Ruan, J.-w., Zeng, Y.-s., Zhou, X., Ding, Y., & Zhou, G.-h. (2015). Improvement in acupoint selection for acupuncture of nerves surrounding the injury site: Electro-acupuncture with Governor vessel with local meridian acupoints. *Neural Regeneration Research, 10,* 128–135. http://dx.doi.org/10.4103/1673-5374.150720

Heinlein, R. A. (1961). *Stranger in a strange land.* New York, NY: Putnam.

Henry, J. A., & Rella, J. G. (2001). Medical risks associated with MDMA use. In J. Holland (Ed.), *Ecstasy: The complete guide—A comprehensive look at the risks and benefits of MDMA* (pp. 71–86). Rochester, VT: Park Street Press.

Herman, J. L. (1992). *Trauma and recovery.* New York: Basic Books.

Hilton, L., Maher, A. R., Colaiaco, B., Apaydin, E., Sorbero, M. E., Booth, M., . . . Hempel, S. (2017). Meditation for posttraumatic stress: Systematic review and meta-analysis. *Psychological Trauma: Theory, Research, Practice, and Policy, 9,* 453–460. http://dx.doi.org/10.1037/tra0000180

Hoge, C. W. (2011). Interventions for war-related posttraumatic stress disorder: Meeting veterans where they are. *JAMA, 306,* 549–551. http://dx.doi.org/10.1001/jama.2011.1096

Hoge, C. W., Castro, C. A., Messer, S. C., McGurk, D., Cotting, D. I., & Koffman, R. L. (2004). Combat duty in Iraq and Afghanistan, mental health problems, and barriers to care. *New England Journal of Medicine, 351,* 13–22. http://dx.doi.org/10.1056/NEJMoa040603

Holland, J. (2001). Medicine for the new millennium. In J. Holland (Ed.), *Ecstasy: A complete guide—A comprehensive look at the risks and benefits of MDMA* (pp. 1–5). Rochester, VT: Park Street Press.

Hollifield, M. (2011). Acupuncture for posttraumatic stress disorder: Conceptual, clinical, and biological data support further research. *CNS Neuroscience & Therapeutics, 17,* 769–779. http://dx.doi.org/10.1111/j.1755-5949.2011.00241.x

Hollifield, M., Sinclair-Lian, N., Warner, T. D., & Hammerschlag, R. (2007). Acupuncture for posttraumatic stress disorder: A randomized controlled pilot trial. *Journal of Nervous and Mental Disease, 195,* 504–513. http://dx.doi.org/10.1097/NMD.0b013e31803044f8

Horn, A., Ostwald, D., Reisert, M., & Blankenburg, F. (2014). The structural–functional connectome and the default mode network of the human brain. *NeuroImage, 102,* 142–151. http://dx.doi.org/10.1016/j.neuroimage.2013.09.069

Horowitz, M., Wilner, N., & Alvarez, W. (1979). Impact of Event Scale: A measure of subjective stress. *Psychosomatic Medicine, 41,* 209–218.

How to begin naming. (n.d.). Retrieved from https://jackkornfield.com/how-to-begin-naming/

Huck, L. G., & Burke, R. L. (2019). *Military veterinary services.* Fort Sam Houston, TX: Office of the Surgeon General, Borden Institute, U.S. Army Medical Department Center and School, Health Readiness Center of Excellence.

Imel, Z. E., Laska, K., Jakupcak, M., & Simpson, T. L. (2013). Meta-analysis of dropout in treatments for posttraumatic stress disorder. *Journal of Consulting and Clinical Psychology, 81,* 394–404. http://dx.doi.org/10.1037/a0031474

Jackson, K. (2014). Treatments for veterans with PTSD—Outside the traditional toolbox. *Social Work Today, 14,* 18. Retrieved from https://www.socialworktoday.com/archive/031714p18.shtml

Jacobson, E. (1938). *Progressive muscle relaxation.* Chicago, IL: University of Chicago Press.

Jaslow, R. (2013, December 26). Common arthroscopic knee surgery no better than "sham" version, researchers say. *CBS News.* Retrieved from https://www.cbsnews.com/news/common-arthroscopic-knee-surgery-not-effective-no-better-than-sham-researchers-say/

Johnson, R. A., Albright, D. L., Marzolf, J. R., Bibbo, J. L., Yaglom, H. D., Crowder, S. M., . . . Harms, N. (2018). Effects of therapeutic horseback riding on post-traumatic stress disorder in military veterans. *Military Medical Research, 5,* 3. http://dx.doi.org/10.1186/s40779-018-0149-6

Jon Kabat-Zinn. (n.d.). In *Wikipedia.* Retrieved from https://en.wikipedia.org/wiki/Jon_Kabat-Zinn

Kabat-Zinn, J. (1990). *Full catastrophe living: Using the wisdom of your body and mind to face stress, pain, and illness.* New York, NY: Bantam Dell.

Kabat-Zinn, J. (1994). *Wherever you go, there you are: Mindfulness meditation in everyday life.* New York, NY: Hyperion.

Kabat-Zinn, J. (2005). *Coming to our senses: Healing ourselves and the world through mindfulness.* New York, NY: Hyperion.

Kaley-Isley, L. C., Peterson, J., Fischer, C., & Peterson, E. (2010). Yoga as complementary therapy for children and adolescents: A guide for clinicians. *Psychiatry, 7,* 20–32.

Keller, S. M., Zoellner, L. A., & Feeny, N. C. (2010). Understanding factors associated with early therapeutic alliance in PTSD treatment: Adherence, childhood sexual abuse history, and social support. *Journal of Consulting and Clinical Psychology, 78,* 974–979. http://dx.doi.org/10.1037/a0020758

Kim, S. H., Schneider, S. M., Kravitz, L., Mermier, C., & Burge, M. R. (2013). Mind-body practices for posttraumatic stress disorder. *Journal of Investigative Medicine, 61,* 827–834. http://dx.doi.org/10.2310/JIM.0b013e3182906862

Kimerling, R. (2004). An investigation of sex differences in nonpsychiatric morbidity associated with posttraumatic stress disorder. *Journal of the American Medical Women's Association, 59,* 43–47.

Kinzie, J. D., Sack, W., Angell, R., Clarke, G., & Ben, R. (1989). A three-year follow-up of Cambodian young people traumatized as children. *Journal of the*

American Academy of Child & Adolescent Psychiatry, 28, 501–504. http://dx.doi.org/10.1097/00004583-198907000-00006

Krystal, H., & Krystal, J. H. (1988). *Integration and self-healing: Affect, trauma, alexithymia.* New York, NY: Analytic Press.

Lachenmeier, D. W., & Rehm, J. (2015). Comparative risk assessment of alcohol, tobacco, cannabis and other illicit drugs using the margin of exposure approach. *Scientific Reports, 5,* Article No. 8126.

Langer, E. J. (2014). *Mindfulness: 25th anniversary edition.* Philadelphia, PA: Da Capo Press.

Lanius, R. A., Bluhm, R., Lanius, U., & Pain, C. (2006). A review of neuroimaging studies in PTSD: Heterogeneity of response to symptom provocation. *Journal of Psychiatric Research, 40,* 709–729. http://dx.doi.org/10.1016/j.jpsychires.2005.07.007

Lanning, B. A., Wilson, A. L., Woelk, R., & Beaujean, A. A. (2018). Therapeutic horseback riding as a complementary intervention for military service members with PTSD. *Human–Animal Interaction Bulletin, 6*(2), 58–82.

Leichsenring, F., & Steinert, C. (2017). Is cognitive behavioral therapy the gold standard for psychotherapy? The need for plurality in treatment and research. *JAMA, 318,* 1323–1324. http://dx.doi.org/10.1001/jama.2017.13737

Lembrou, P. T., Pratt, G. J., & Chevalier, G. (2003). Physiological and psychological effects of mind/body therapy on claustrophobia. *Subtle Energies & Energy Medicine, 14*(1), 239–251.

Levine, P. (2010). *In an unspoken voice: How the body releases trauma and restores goodness.* Berkeley, CA: North Atlantic Books.

Libby, D. J., Pilver, C. E., & Desai, R. (2012). Complementary and alternative medicine in VA specialized PTSD treatment programs. *Psychiatric Services, 63,* 1134–1136. http://dx.doi.org/10.1176/appi.ps.201100456

Lin, T.-W., & Kuo, Y.-M. (2013). Exercise benefits brain function: The monoamine connection. *Brain Sciences, 3*(1), 39–53. http://dx.doi.org/10.3390/brainsci3010039

Linehan, M. M. (1993). *Cognitive behavioral treatment for borderline personality disorder.* New York, NY: Guilford Press.

Lupien, S. J., McEwen, B. S., Gunnar, M. R., & Heim, C. (2009). Effects of stress throughout the lifespan on the brain, behaviour and cognition. *Nature Reviews Neuroscience, 10,* 434–445. http://dx.doi.org/10.1038/nrn2639

Lynch, J. H., Mulvaney, S. W., Kim, E. H., de Leeuw, J. B., Schroeder, M. J., & Kane, S. F. (2016). Effect of stellate ganglion block on specific symptom clusters for treatment of post-traumatic stress disorder. *Military Medicine, 181,* 1135–1141. http://dx.doi.org/10.7205/MILMED-D-15-00518

MacPherson, H., Vickers, A., Bland, M., Torgerson, D., Corbett, M., Spackman, E., . . . Watt, I. (2017). Acupuncture for chronic pain and depression in primary care: A programme of research. *Programme Grants for Applied Research, 5*(3), 1–316.

Manger, T. A., & Motta, R. W. (2005). The impact of an exercise program on posttraumatic stress disorder, anxiety, and depression. *International Journal of Emergency Mental Health, 7,* 49–57.

Marich, J. (2011). *EMDR made simple: 4 approaches to using EMDR with every client.* Eau Claire, WI: Premier.

Martin, D. P., Sletten, C. D., Williams, B. A., & Berger, I. H. (2006). Improvement in fibromyalgia symptoms with acupuncture: Results of a randomized controlled trial. *Mayo Clinic Proceedings, 81,* 749–757. http://dx.doi.org/10.4065/81.6.749

McCann, I. L., & Pearlman, L. A. (1990). Vicarious traumatisation: A framework for understanding the psychological effects of working with victims. *Journal of Traumatic Stress, 3*, 131–149.

McNally, R. J. (1999). Research on eye movement desensitization and reprocessing (EMDR) as a treatment for PTSD. *PTSD Research Quarterly, 10*, 1–2.

Mead, E. (2020, January 17). *The history and origin of meditation.* Retrieved from https://positivepsychology.com/history-of-meditation/

Mens sana in corpore sano [A healthy mind in a healthy body]. (n.d.). In *Wikipedia.* Retrieved from https://en.wikipedia.org/wiki/Mens_sana_in_corpore_sano

Meta-analysis of dropout in treatments for posttraumatic stress disorder: Correction to Imel et al. (2013). (2016). *Journal of Consulting and Clinical Psychology, 84*, 838.

Miller, R. C. (2007). *Integrative restoration: Level I training manual.* Larkspur, CA: Integrative Restoration Institute.

Miller, R. C. (2015). *The iRest program for healing PTSD: A proven-effective approach to using yoga nidra meditation & deep relaxation techniques to overcome trauma.* Oakland, CA: New Harbinger.

Mithoefer, M. C. (2017). *A manual for MDMA-assisted psychotherapy in the treatment of posttraumatic stress disorder* (Version 8.1). Santa Cruz, CA: Multidisciplinary Association for Psychedelic Studies. Retrieved from https://s3-us-west-1.amazonaws.com/mapscontent/research-archive/mdma/TreatmentManual_MDMAAssistedPsychotherapyVersion+8.1_22+Aug2017.pdf

Mithoefer, M. C., Wagner, M. T., Mithoefer, A. T., Jerome, L., & Doblin, R. (2011). The safety and efficacy of ± 3,4-methylenedioxymethamphetamine-assisted psychotherapy in subjects with chronic, treatment-resistant posttraumatic stress disorder: The first randomized controlled pilot study. *Journal of Psychopharmacology, 25*, 439–452. http://dx.doi.org/10.1177/0269881110378371

Mithoefer, M. C., Wagner, M. T., Mithoefer, A. T., Jerome, L., Martin, S. F., Yazar-Klosinski, B., . . . Doblin, R. (2013). Durability of improvement in post-traumatic stress disorder symptoms and absence of harmful effects of drug dependency after 3,4-methylenedioxymethamphetamine-assisted psychotherapy: A prospective long-term follow-up study. *Journal of Psychopharmacology, 27*, 28–39. http://dx.doi.org/10.1177/0269881112456611

Morina, N., Wicherts, J. M., Lobbrecht, J., & Priebe, S. (2014). Remission from post-traumatic stress disorder in adults: A systematic review and meta-analysis of long-term outcome studies. *Clinical Psychology Review, 34*, 249–255. http://dx.doi.org/10.1016/j.cpr.2014.03.002

Morris, D. J. (2015). *The evil hours: A biography of post-traumatic stress disorder.* New York, NY: Houghton Mifflin Harcourt.

Motta, R. W. (2008). Secondary trauma. *International Journal of Emergency Mental Health, 10*, 291–298.

Motta, R. W. (2013, Winter). PTSD and secondary traumatization: A comprehensive review. *Mental Health News*, pp. 1, 6, 14, 16, 22, 26, 27, 30. Retrieved from http://mhnews.org/back_issues/MHN-Winter2013.pdf

Motta, R. W. (2015). Trauma, PTSD, and secondary trauma in children and adolescents. In R. Flanagan (Ed.), *Cognitive and behavioral interventions in the schools* (pp. 67–84). New York, NY: Springer. http://dx.doi.org/10.1007/978-1-4939-1972-7_4

Motta, R. W. (2018a, Summer). The role of exercise in alleviating anxiety, depression, and PTSD. *Behavioral Health News*, pp. 33, 37. Retrieved from http://mhnews.org/back_issues/BHN-Summer2018.pdf

Motta, R. W. (2018b). The role of exercise in reducing PTSD and negative emotional states. In S. G. Taukeni (Ed.), *Psychology of health—Biopsychosocial approach.* http://dx.doi.org/10.5772/intechopen.81012

Motta, R., & Lynch, C. (1990). Therapeutic techniques vs therapeutic relationships in child behavior therapy. *Psychological Reports, 67,* 315–322. http://dx.doi.org/10.2466%2Fpr0.1990.67.1.315

Motta, R. W., McWilliams, M. E., Schwartz, J. T., & Cavera, R. S. (2012). The role of exercise in reducing childhood and adolescent PTSD, anxiety, and depression. *Journal of Applied School Psychology, 28,* 224–238. http://dx.doi.org/10.1080/15377903.2012.695765

Mulcahy, K. A. (1998). *Beck's cognitive therapy and aerobic exercise for the treatment of depression* (Unpublished doctoral dissertation). Hofstra University, Hempstead, NY.

Multidisciplinary Association for Psychedelic Studies. (n.d.). MDMA-assisted psychotherapy study protocols [Research]. Retrieved from https://maps.org/research/mdma

Multidisciplinary Association for Psychedelic Studies. (2014a, January 26). *A manual for MDMA-assisted psychotherapy in the treatment of PTSD.* Retrieved from https://maps.org/research/mdma/mdma-research-timeline/4887-a-manual-for-mdma-assisted-psychotherapy-in-the-treatment-of-ptsd

Multidisciplinary Association for Psychedelic Studies. (2014b, December 16). *MAPS receives $2 million grant from Colorado for study of medical marijuana for PTSD* [Press release]. Retrieved from https://maps.org/news/media/5445-press-release-maps-receives-$2-million-grant-from-colorado-for-study-of-medical-marijuana-for-ptsd

National Institute of Mental Health. (2000). *Depression in children and adolescents* (Fact sheet for physicians; NIH Publication No. 00-4744). Bethesda, MD: Author.

National Institute on Drug Abuse. (n.d.). *What is the history of MDMA?* Retrieved from https://www.drugabuse.gov/publications/research-reports/mdma-ecstasy-abuse/what-is-the-history-of-mdma

National Psychologist Staff. (2016, July 27). *SAMHSA adds thought field therapy to National Registry.* Retrieved from https://nationalpsychologist.com/2016/07/samhsa-adds-thought-field-therapy-to-national-registry/103335.html

Neill, J. T. (2003). Reviewing and benchmarking adventure therapy outcomes: Applications of meta-analysis. *Journal of Experiential Education, 25,* 316–321. http://dx.doi.org/10.1177/105382590302500305

Neria, Y., Nandi, A., & Galea, S. (2008). Post-traumatic stress disorder following disasters: A systematic review. *Psychological Medicine, 38,* 467–480. http://dx.doi.org/10.1017/S0033291707001353

Newman, C. L., & Motta, R. W. (2007). The effects of aerobic exercise on childhood PTSD, anxiety, and depression. *International Journal of Emergency Mental Health, 9,* 133–158.

Nichols, D. E. (1986). Differences between the mechanism of action of MDMA, MBDB, and the classic hallucinogens. Identification of a new therapeutic class: Entactogens. *Journal of Psychoactive Drugs, 18,* 305–313. http://dx.doi.org/10.1080/02791072.1986.10472362

Nightingale, F. (1969). *Notes on nursing: What it is, and what it is not.* New York, NY: Dover.

Nisbet, M. (2017, May/June). The mindfulness movement: How a Buddhist practice evolved into a scientific approach to life. *Skeptical Inquirer, 41*(3), 24–26.

Norris, R., Carroll, D., & Cochrane, R. (1992). The effects of physical activity and exercise training on psychological stress and well-being in an adolescent population. *Journal of Psychosomatic Research, 36,* 55–65. http://dx.doi.org/10.1016/0022-3999(92)90114-H

Oehen, P., Traber, R., Widmer, V., & Schnyder, U. (2013). A randomized, controlled pilot study of MDMA (3,4-methylenedioxymethamphetamine)-assisted psychotherapy for treatment of resistant, chronic post-traumatic stress disorder (PTSD). *Journal of Psychopharmacology, 27,* 40–52. http://dx.doi.org/10.1177/0269881112464827

O'Haire, M. E., & Rodriguez, K. E. (2018). Preliminary efficacy of service dogs as a complementary treatment for posttraumatic stress disorder in military members and veterans. *Journal of Consulting and Clinical Psychology, 86,* 179–188. http://dx.doi.org/10.1037/ccp0000267

Ortner, N. (2013). *The tapping solution: A revolutionary system for stress-free living.* New York, NY: Hay House.

Ortner, N. (2015). *The tapping solution for pain relief: A step-by-step guide to reducing and eliminating chronic pain.* New York, NY: Hay House.

Paluska, S. A., & Schwenk, T. L. (2000). Physical activity and mental health: Current concepts. *Sports Medicine, 29,* 167–180. http://dx.doi.org/10.2165/00007256-200029030-00003

Parfitt, G., & Eston, R. G. (2005). The relationship between children's habitual activity level and psychological well-being. *Acta Paediatrica, 94,* 1791–1797. http://dx.doi.org/10.1111/j.1651-2227.2005.tb01855.x

Parish-Plass, N. (2008). Animal-assisted therapy with children suffering from insecure attachment due to abuse and neglect: A method to lower the risk of intergenerational transmission of abuse? *Clinical Child Psychology and Psychiatry, 13,* 7–30. http://dx.doi.org/10.1177/1359104507086338

Patki, G., Li, L., Allam, F., Solanki, N., Dao, A. T., Alkadhi, K., & Salim, S. (2014). Moderate treadmill exercise rescues anxiety and depression-like behavior as well as memory impairment in a rat model of posttraumatic stress disorder. *Physiology & Behavior, 130,* 47–53. http://dx.doi.org/10.1016/j.physbeh.2014.03.016

Peluso, M. A. M., & Guerra de Andrade, L. H. S. (2005). Physical activity and mental health: The association between exercise and mood. *Clinics, 60,* 61–70. http://dx.doi.org/10.1590/S1807-59322005000100012

Pendry, P., Smith, A. N., & Roeter, S. M. (2014). Randomized trial examines effects of equine facilitated learning on adolescents' basal cortisol levels. *Human–Animal Interaction Bulletin, 2*(1), 80–95.

Pert, C. B. (1999). *Molecules of emotion: The science behind mind-body medicine.* New York, NY: Scribner.

Pet Partners. (n.d.). *Terminology: Industry terms.* Retrieved from https://petpartners.org/learn/terminology/

Pomeranz, B. (1989). Acupuncture analgesia for chronic pain: Brief survey of clinical trials. In B. Pomeranx & G. Stux (Eds.), *Scientific bases of acupuncture* (pp. 197–199). Berlin, Germany: Springer-Verlag. http://dx.doi.org/10.1007/978-3-642-73757-2_11

Poulsen, D. V., Stigsdotter, U. K., & Refshage, A. D. (2015). Whatever happened to the soldiers? Nature-assisted therapies for veterans diagnosed with post-traumatic stress disorder: A literature review. *Urban Forestry & Urban Greening, 14,* 438–445. http://dx.doi.org/10.1016/j.ufug.2015.03.009

Preston, J. D., O'Neal, J. H., & Talaga, M. C. (2002). *Handbook of clinical psychopharmacology for therapists* (3rd ed.). Oakland, CA: New Harbinger.

Reinhardt, K. M., Noggle Taylor, J. J., Johnston, J., Zameer, A., Cheema, S., & Khalsa, S. B. S. (2018). Kripalu yoga for military veterans with PTSD: A randomized trial. *Journal of Clinical Psychology, 74,* 93–108. http://dx.doi.org/10.1002/jclp.22483

Relf, P. D. (2005). The therapeutic values of plants. *Pediatric Rehabilitation, 8,* 235–237. http://dx.doi.org/10.1080/13638490400011140

Resick, P. A. (2001). *Cognitive processing therapy: Generic version.* St Louis: University of Missouri-St. Louis.

Reynolds, C. R., & Richmond, B. O. (1985). *Revised children's manifest anxiety scale.* Los Angeles, CA: Western Psychological Services.

Rhodes, A., Spinazzola, J., & van der Kolk, B. (2016). Yoga for adult women with chronic PTSD: A long-term follow-up study. *Journal of Alternative and Complementary Medicine, 22,* 189–196. http://dx.doi.org/10.1089/acm.2014.0407

Riley, K. E., & Park, C. L. (2015). How does yoga reduce stress? A systematic review of mechanisms of change and guide to future inquiry. *Health Psychology Review, 9,* 379–396. http://dx.doi.org/10.1080/17437199.2014.981778

Robotti, S. B. (2019, August 24). *Drug classifications, Schedule I, II, III, IV, V.* Retrieved from https://medshadow.org/drug-classifications-schedule-ii-iii-iv-v/

Rodriguez, N., Ryan, S. W., Rowan, A. B., & Foy, D. W. (1996). Posttraumatic stress disorder in a clinical sample of adult survivors of childhood sexual abuse. *Child Abuse & Neglect, 20,* 943–952. http://dx.doi.org/10.1016/0145-2134(96)00083-X

Rogers, S., & Silver, S. M. (2002). Is EMDR an exposure therapy? A review of trauma protocols. *Journal of Clinical Psychology, 58,* 43–59. http://dx.doi.org/10.1002/jclp.1128

Rohleder, N., & Karl, A. (2006). Role of endocrine and inflammatory alterations in comorbid somatic diseases of post-traumatic stress disorder. *Minerva Endocrinologica, 31,* 273–288.

Rothbaum, B. O. (1997). A controlled study of eye movement desensitization and reprocessing in the treatment of posttraumatic stress disordered sexual assault victims. *Bulletin of the Menninger Clinic, 61,* 317–334.

Rothbaum, B. O., Astin, M. C., & Marsteller, F. (2005). Prolonged exposure versus eye movement desensitization and reprocessing (EMDR) for PTSD in rape victims. *Journal of Traumatic Stress, 18,* 607–616. http://dx.doi.org/10.1002/jts.20069

Rozak, R. (1993). *The voice of the earth.* New York, NY: Simon & Schuster.

Salzberg, S. (1995). *Lovingkindness: The revolutionary art of happiness.* Boston, MA: Shambhala.

Schnurr, P. P., Friedman, M. J., Foy, D. W., Shea, M. T., Hsieh, F. Y., Lavori, P. W., . . . Bernardy, N. C. (2003). Randomized trial of trauma-focused group therapy for posttraumatic stress disorder: Results from a Department of Veterans Affairs cooperative study. *Archives of General Psychiatry, 60,* 481–489. http://dx.doi.org/10.1001/archpsyc.60.5.481

Schottenbauer, M. A., Glass, C. R., Arnkoff, D. B., Tendick, V., & Gray, S. H. (2008). Nonresponse and dropout rates in outcome studies on PTSD: Review and methodological considerations. *Psychiatry, 71,* 134–168. http://dx.doi.org/10.1521/psyc.2008.71.2.134

Sebastian, B., & Nelms, J. (2017). The effectiveness of emotional freedom techniques in the treatment of posttraumatic stress disorder: A meta-analysis. *Explore, 13,* 16–25. http://dx.doi.org/10.1016/j.explore.2016.10.001

Shapiro, F. (1989). Eye movement desensitization: A new treatment for posttraumatic stress disorder. *Journal of Behavior Therapy and Experimental Psychiatry, 20,* 211–217. http://dx.doi.org/10.1016/0005-7916(89)90025-6

Shapiro, F. (2001). *Eye movement desensitization and reprocessing: Basic principles, protocols and procedures* (2nd ed.). New York, NY: Guilford Press.

Shen, J., Wenger, N., Glaspy, J., Hays, R. D., Albert, P. S., Choi, C., & Shekelle, P. G. (2000). Electroacupuncture for control of myeloablative chemotherapy-induced emesis: A randomized controlled trial. *JAMA, 284,* 2755–2761. http://dx.doi.org/10.1001/jama.284.21.2755

Shin, L. M., Orr, S. P., Carson, M. A., Rauch, S. L., Macklin, M. L., Lasko, N. B., . . . Pitman, R. K. (2004). Regional cerebral blood flow in the amygdala and medial prefrontal cortex during traumatic imagery in male and female Vietnam veterans with PTSD. *Archives of General Psychiatry, 61,* 168–176. http://dx.doi.org/10.1001/archpsyc.61.2.168

Shivakumar, G., Anderson, E. H., Surís, A. M., & North, C. S. (2017). Exercise for PTSD in women veterans: A proof-of-concept study. *Military Medicine, 182,* e1809–e1814. http://dx.doi.org/10.7205/MILMED-D-16-00440

Sihvonen, R., Paavola, M., Malmivaara, A., Itälä, A., Joukainen, A., Nurmi, H., . . . Järvinen, T. L. N. (2013). Arthroscopic partial meniscectomy versus sham surgery for a degenerative meniscal tear. *The New England Journal of Medicine, 369,* 2515–2524. http://dx.doi.org/10.1056/NEJMoa1305189

Silvestri, L. (2001). Anxiety reduction though aerobic dance and progressive relaxation training. *Education, 108,* 34–40.

Smaga, I., Bystrowska, B., Gawlinski, D., Przegalinski, E., & Filip, M. (2014). The endocannabinoid/endovanilloid system and depression. *Current Neuropharmacology, 12,* 462–474. http://dx.doi.org/10.2174/1570159X12666140923205412

Sobo, E. J., Eng, B., & Kassity-Krich, N. (2006). Canine visitation (pet) therapy: Pilot data on decreases in child pain perception. *Journal of Holistic Nursing, 24,* 51–57.

Soler, J., Cebolla, A., Feliu-Soler, A., Demarzo, M. M. P., Pascual, J. C., Baños, R., & García-Campayo, J. (2014). Relationship between meditative practice and self-reported mindfulness: The MINDSENS composite index. *PLOS ONE, 9,* e86622. http://dx.doi.org/10.1371/journal.pone.0086622

Stein, P. N., & Motta, R. W. (1992). Effects of aerobic and nonaerobic exercise on depression and self-concept. *Perceptual and Motor Skills, 74,* 79–89. http://dx.doi.org/10.2466/pms.1992.74.1.79

Stickgold, R. (2002). EMDR: A putative neurobiological mechanism of action. *Journal of Clinical Psychology, 58,* 61–75. http://dx.doi.org/10.1002/jclp.1129

Strauss, J. L., Coeytaux, R., McDuffie, J., & Williams, J. W., Jr. (2011, August). *Efficacy of complementary and alternative medicine therapies for posttraumatic stress disorder* (VA-ESP Project No. 09-010). Washington, DC: Department of Veterans Affairs, Health Services Research & Development Service. Retrieved from http://atthespeedofsight.com/wellnessembassy/pdfs/Efficacy_of_CAM_for_PTSD_VA.pdf

Su, D., & Li, L. (2011). Trends in the use of complementary and alternative medicine in the United States: 2002–2007. *Journal of Health Care for the Poor and Underserved, 22,* 296–310.

Sun, H., Zhao, H., Ma, C., Bao, F., Zhang, J., Wang, D.-h., . . . He, W. (2013). Effects of electroacupuncture on depression and the production of glial cell line-derived neurotrophic factor compared with fluoxetine: A randomized controlled pilot study. *Journal of Alternative and Complementary Medicine, 19,* 733–739. http://dx.doi.org/10.1089/acm.2011.0637

Swingle, P. G., Pulos, L., & Swingle, M. K. (2003). Neurophysiological indicators of EFT treatment of post-traumatic stress. *Subtle Energies & Energy Medicine, 15*(1), 75–86.

Synovitz, L. B., & Larson, K. L. (2013). *Complementary and alternative medicine for health professionals: A holistic approach to consumer health.* Burlington, MA: Jones & Bartlett Learning.

Teasdale, J. D., Segal, Z. V., Williams, J. M., Ridgeway, V. A., Soulsby, J. M., & Lau, M. A. (2000). Prevention of relapse/recurrence in major depression by mindfulness-based cognitive therapy. *Journal of Consulting and Clinical Psychology, 68,* 615–623. http://dx.doi.org/10.1037/0022-006X.68.4.615

The Tapping Solution: Documentary Film on EFT Tapping [YouTube video]. (2008, September 16). Retrieved from https://www.youtube.com/watch?v=vzE0ZvMM3gM

Thibault, R. T., & Raz, A. (2017). The psychology of neurofeedback: Clinical intervention even if applied placebo. *American Psychologist, 72,* 679–688. http://dx.doi.org/10.1037/amp0000118

Treleaven, D. A. (2018). *Trauma-sensitive mindfulness: Practices for safe and transformative healing.* New York, NY: Norton.

Trimble, M. R. (1981). *Post-traumatic neurosis. From railway spine to whiplash.* New York, NY: Wiley.

Trimble, M. R. (1985). Post-traumatic stress disorder: History of a concept. In C. R. Figley (Ed.), *Trauma and its wake: The study and treatment of post-traumatic stress disorder* (pp. 5–14). New York, NY: Bruner/Mazel.

Turow, R. G. (2017). *Mindfulness skills for trauma and PTSD.* New York, NY: Norton.

U.S. Department of Veterans Affairs & U.S. Department of Defense. (2017, June). *VA/DOD clinical practice guideline for the management of posttraumatic stress disorder and acute stress disorder.* Retrieved from https://www.healthquality.va.gov/guidelines/MH/ptsd/VADoDPTSDCPGFinal010818.pdf

van der Kolk, B. A. (2005). Developmental trauma disorder: Toward a rational diagnosis for children with complex trauma histories. *Psychiatric Annals, 35,* 401–408. http://dx.doi.org/10.3928/00485713-20050501-06

van der Kolk, B. A. (2006). Clinical implications of neuroscience research in PTSD. *Annals of the New York Academy of Sciences, 1071,* 277–293. http://dx.doi.org/10.1196/annals.1364.022

van der Kolk, B. A. (2014). *The body keeps the score: Brain, mind, and body in the healing of trauma.* New York, NY: Viking.

van der Kolk, B. A., Stone, L., West, J., Rhodes, A., Emerson, D., Suvak, M., & Spinazzola, J. (2014). Yoga as an adjunctive treatment for posttraumatic stress disorder: A randomized controlled trial. *Journal of Clinical Psychiatry, 75,* e559–e565. http://dx.doi.org/10.4088/JCP.13m08561

Varvogli, L., & Darviri, C. (2011). Stress management techniques: Evidence-based procedures that reduce stress and promote health. *Health Science Journal, 5,* 74–89.

Vickers, A. J., Cronin, A. M., Maschino, A. C., Lewith, G., MacPherson, H., Foster, N. E., . . . Linde, K. (2012). Acupuncture for chronic pain: Individual patient data meta-analysis. *Archives of Internal Medicine, 172,* 1444–1453. http://dx.doi.org/10.1001/archinternmed.2012.3654

Vujanovic, A. A., Niles, B., Pietrefesa, A., Schmertz, S. K., & Potter, C. M. (2013). Mindfulness in the treatment of posttraumatic stress disorder among military veterans. *Spirituality in Clinical Practice, 1,* 15–25. http://dx.doi.org/10.1037/2326-4500.1.S.15

Waddell, C., & Godderis, R. (2005). Rethinking evidence-based practice for children's mental health. *Evidence-Based Mental Health, 8,* 60–62. http://dx.doi.org/10.1136/ebmh.8.3.60

Wampold, B. E. (2015). How important are the common factors in psychotherapy? An update. *World Psychiatry, 14,* 270–277. http://dx.doi.org/10.1002/wps.20238

Wampold, B. E., Imel, Z. E., Laska, K. M., Benish, S., Miller, S. D., Flückiger, C., . . . Budge, S. (2010). Determining what works in the treatment of PTSD. *Clinical Psychology Review, 30,* 923–933. http://dx.doi.org/10.1016/j.cpr.2010.06.005

Watson, S. (n.d.). *Acupuncture overview: The history of acupuncture.* Retrieved from https://health.howstuffworks.com/wellness/natural-medicine/alternative/acupuncture6.htm

Weintraub, A. (2012). *Yoga skills for therapists: Effective practices for mood management.* New York, NY: Norton.

Whitworth, J. W., Craft, L. L., Dunsiger, S. I., & Ciccolo, J. T. (2017). Direct and indirect effects of exercise on posttraumatic stress disorder symptoms: A longitudinal study. *General Hospital Psychiatry, 49,* 56–62. http://dx.doi.org/10.1016/j.genhosppsych.2017.06.012

Williams, F. (2017). *The nature fix.* New York, NY: Norton.

Wilson, E. O. (1984). *Biophilia.* Cambridge, MA: Harvard University Press.

Wolpe, J., & Lazarus, A. A. (1966). *Behavior therapy techniques: A guide to the treatment of neuroses.* Elmsford, NY: Pergamon Press.

World Health Organization. (2002). *Acupuncture: Review and analysis of reports on controlled clinical trials.* Geneva, Switzerland: Author.

World Health Organization. (2013, August 6). *WHO releases guidance on mental health care after trauma* [Press release]. Retrieved from https://www.who.int/mediacentre/news/releases/2013/trauma_mental_health_20130806/en/

World Health Organization. (2018). *International classification of diseases for mortality and morbidity statistics* (11th revision). Geneva, Switzerland: Author.

Wright, R. (2017). *Why Buddhism is true: The science and philosophy of meditation and enlightenment.* New York, NY: Simon & Schuster.

Yarborough, B. J. H., Stumbo, S. P., Yarborough, M. T., Owen-Smith, A., & Green, C. A. (2018). Benefits and challenges of using service dogs for veterans with posttraumatic stress disorder. *Psychiatric Rehabilitation Journal, 41,* 118–124. http://dx.doi.org/10.1037/prj0000294

Yasinski, C., Hayes, A. M., Alpert, E., McCauley, T., Ready, C. B., Webb, C., & Deblinger, E. (2018). Treatment processes and demographic variables as predictors of dropout from trauma-focused cognitive behavioral therapy (TF-CBT) for youth. *Behaviour Research and Therapy, 107,* 10–18. http://dx.doi.org/10.1016/j.brat.2018.05.008

Yehuda, R., & LeDoux, J. (2007). Response variation following trauma: A translational neuroscience approach to understanding PTSD. *Neuron, 56*, 19–32. http://dx.doi.org/10.1016/j.neuron.2007.09.006

Zayfert, C., Deviva, J. C., Becker, C. B., Pike, J. L., Gillock, K. L., & Hayes, S. A. (2005). Exposure utilization and completion of cognitive behavioral therapy for PTSD in a "real world" clinical practice. *Journal of Traumatic Stress, 18*, 637–645. http://dx.doi.org/10.1002/jts.20072

Zhang, R., Feng, X.-J., Guan, Q., Cui, W., Zheng, Y., Sun, W., & Han, J.-S. (2011). Increase of success rate for women undergoing embryo transfer by transcutaneous electrical acupoint stimulation: A prospective randomized placebo-controlled study. *Fertility and Sterility, 96*, 912–916. http://dx.doi.org/10.1016/j.fertnstert.2011.07.1093

INDEX

ABOUT THE AUTHOR

Robert W. Motta, PhD, ABPP, is a professor of psychology and director of the doctoral program in School-Community Psychology at Hofstra University in New York. He is also the director of Hofstra's Child and Family Trauma Institute. Formerly, he was the chair of the psychology department. Dr. Motta served in the U.S. Army's 1st Cavalry Division during the Vietnam War and is board certified in both cognitive behavior psychology and behavioral psychology. He has published more than 100 scientific papers, primarily in refereed psychology journals. He is also on the examining board of the American Board of Professional Psychology and is a licensed clinical psychologist, certified school psychologist, and past president and secretary–treasurer of the School Psychology division of the New York State Psychological Association.